How to have Sound Sleep
—the natural way

Dr. A.K. Sethi
(M.B.B.S., F.C.C.P.)

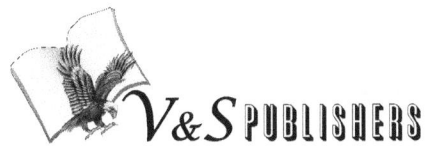

Published by:

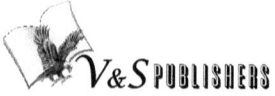

F-2/16, Ansari Road, Daryaganj, New Delhi-110002
☎ 011-23240026, 011-23240027 • *Fax:* 011-23240028
Email: info@vspublishers.com • *Website:* www.vspublishers.com

Branch: Hyderabad
5-1-707/1, Brij Bhawan (Beside Central Bank of India Lane)
Bank Street, Koti Hyderabad - 500 095
☎ 040-24737290
E-mail: vspublishershyd@gmail.com

Distributors:

▶ **Pustak Mahal®**, Delhi
J-3/16, Daryaganj, New Delhi-110002
☎ 011-23276539, 011-23272783, 011-23272784 • *Fax:* 011-23260518
E-mail: sales@pustakmahal.com • *Website:* www.pustakmahal.com
Bengaluru: ☎ 080-22234025 • *Telefax:* 080-22240209
Patna: ☎ 0612-3294193 • *Telefax:* 0612-2302719

▶ **PM Publications**
- 10-B, Netaji Subhash Marg, Daryaganj, New Delhi-110002
  ☎ 011-23268292, 011-23268293, 011-23279900 • *Fax:* 011-23280567
  E-mail: pmpublications@gmail.com
- 6686, Khari Baoli, Delhi-110006
  ☎ 011-23944314, 011-23911979

▶ **Unicorn Books**
Mumbai:
23-25, Zaoba Wadi (Opp. VIP Showroom), Thakurdwar, Mumbai-400002
☎ 022-22010941 • *Telefax:* 022-22053387

© Copyright: V&S PUBLISHERS
ISBN 978-93-813849-7-8
Edition: 2011

The Copyright of this book, as well as all matters contained herein (including illustrations) rests with the Publisher. No person shall copy the name of the book, its title design, matter and illustrations in any form and in any language, totally or partially or in any form. Anybody doing so shall face legal action and will be responsible for damages.

Printed at: Unique Colour Carton, Mayapuri

Preface

Getting sound sleep is as essential as food and water for well-being of mind and body. It is the most precious commodity capable of providing rest and nourishment to a tired brain and body. In today's fast and strenuous life, it has become difficult to follow a strict pattern of going to bed at a fixed time and then falling off into deep sleep promptly.

Due to hectic pace of life, sleep disorders are spreading fast. People are worried about the adverse effects on their health. They are anxious to know the kinds of sleep disorders, their causes, and treatment. Due to the addictive and harmful effects of sleeping pills, interest is growing in the role of Yoga, Naturopathy, Ayurveda, Acupressure, Magnetotherapy, Chromotherapy, Music Therapy, Aromatherapy, Feng Shui and Vaastu Shastra can play in prevention and cure of sleep disorders. I hope readers will find this book useful.

—*Dr. A.K. SETHI*

Acknowledgements

At the outset, I must thank V&S Publishers for giving me the opportunity to write this book for laymen on an ailment which is widely prevalent around the globe. I am also grateful to the patients who came to our clinic with the problems of sleep disorders and benefited from the alternative forms of treatment provided to them. I am indebted to Mr. R. L. Jaggi, retired Senior Accounts Officer (Northern Railways), who has been successfully practising Chromotherapy and provided me with abundant literature on different systems of Alternative Medicine. (Dr.) Swami Ananta Bharati, Chairman and Founder of Swami Keshwananda Yoga Institute, has thoroughly guided me and taught the art of Yoga, Pranayama and Meditation. Mr. N.S. Dabas, an eminent astrologer and Vaastu Shastri, who is a staunch believer, follower and practitioner of Magnetotherapy, also assisted me in these fields. Dr. Ruma Banerjee, a practising Physiotherapist and Naturopath has guided me in her area of expertise.

My wife, Dr. Sunanda Sethi, an Ayurvedacharya and a Traditional Reiki Master, has been a source of inspiration. I thank my children-Rupal and Mitali-without whose cooperation this book would not have been completed.

—Dr. A.K. SETHI

Contents

Preface 3

Acknowledgements 5

1. Sleep 9
2. Physiology of Sleep 15
3. How to Have Sound Sleep 19
4. Sleep Disorders 25
5. Snoring 31
6. Nightmares 36
7. Sleepwalking 38
8. Sleepiness 40
9. Hypersomnia 44
10. How to Tackle Sleep Disorders 44
11. Lifestyle Suggestions to Enhance Sleep 125
12. Recent Advances in Diagnosis Treatment of Sleep Disorders 129

Chapter 1

Sleep

Sleep is one of the most important necessities of life. We spend nearly one-third of our life sleeping. *Shakespeare* has said, "Sleep is the balm of the hurt minds; great nature's second course; chief nourisher in life's feast."

In the words of *Napoleon*, "What a delightful thing rest is! The bed has become a place of luxury to me. I would not exchange it for all the thrones in the world."

It has been said, "Blessing on him who first invented sleep. It covers a man all over, thoughts and all, like a cloak. It is meat for the hungry, drink for the thirsty, heat for the cold and cold for the hot."

The importance of sleep should not be underestimated. It is a "tired nature's sweet restorer" or the most important gift of God.

Why Do We Need Sleep?

There are countless cells in our body which require rest for relaxation and vitality. If not given enough rest, these cells, will tire themselves out and become less functional and erratic. Proper and sound sleep is essential for rejuvenation of heart muscles that get fatigued during the day. The better the quality of sleep, the more rest these cells and tissues get and perform better by making our body carry out the daily routine effectively.

In essence, sleep is a tonic for our physical and mental health. It removes exertion, and imparts our body and mind with freshness, energy and strength. It reinvigorates strained muscles and nerves.

Benefits of Sound Sleep

The benefits desired from a sound sleep are:

1. It gives rest to strained muscles and nerves.
2. It soothes the body, the mind and the soul.
3. It conserves the energy of our body.
4. It enables proper growth in children since the maximum secretion of growth hormone occurs at night.
5. It helps repair the cells and tissues that are damaged due to various illnesses.
6. Regular sleep gives rest to our facial muscles as well as the skin, thus keeping it free from wrinkles.
7. It helps in boosting the immune system which is responsible for defence of the body against illnesses; and their speedy recovery.
8. A sound sleep reduces the day-long fatigue of our body.
9. The physical and mental energy lost during the day is regained during the night.
10. It rejuvenates our body, helping us to face the new day fresh.
11. Medical research has shown that the people who have a regular and adequate sleep do not suffer from heart diseases and hypertension.

12. Sound sleep for at least 6 to 8 hours daily helps to prolong the lifespan of the individuals.
13. Studies have also shown that regular sleeping patterns help in the prevention of many infections and even cancer.

Adverse Effects of Lack of Sleep/ Disturbed Sleep

Modernisation of lifestyle and civilization controls our sleep to a large extent. Inadequate or disturbed sleep can give rise to a number of problems. These problems may be mild when sleep is disturbed only for a day or two but aggravate if disturbed continuously for many nights.

Following problems may arise due to lack of adequate sleep:

1. The person becomes irritable and loses his temper over trivial matters.
2. He may feel restless while sitting, standing or even lying down.
3. He complains of a constant headache especially involving the forehead and eyes.
4. A person with disturbed sleep feels as if his body is aching and finds it uneasy to move around.
5. The most common effect of lack of sleep is fatigue. The person feels tired and complains of lack of energy.
6. The person shows diminished interest in his work and surroundings.
7. It may lead to repeated yawning, dozing off and drowsiness.
8. Depression, anxiety, giddiness and even fits (convulsions) may set in, especially in the people, who are prone to mental illnesses.

9. Many individuals report changes in heartbeat or pulse rate and blood pressure.
10. Researchers have observed that when people don't get enough sleep, their ability to think suffers.
11. Chronic insomnia can impair orientation to time and place, *i.e.* person is not aware of the time and place where he is present.
12. Some individuals develop dark circles under the eyes and a greyish tinge of skin.
13. People with prolonged sleep disorders cannot put forth their best efforts and their performance at work is unsatisfactory.
14. Major industrial and road accidents are usually caused by individuals with sleep disorder.
15. It has been found that those, who have been deprived of adequate sleep for a long time, may develop heart diseases, hypertension, certain infections and even cancer.

The adverse effects of lack of sleep on an individual may be summarised as under:

1. Irritability
2. Restlessness
3. Constant headache
4. Heaviness in the body
5. Fatigue
6. Lack of interest in work
7. Lethargy with yawning, drowsiness, dozing off
8. Depression/anxiety
9. Giddiness
10. Fits
11. Changes in heartbeat and blood pressure
12. Poor memory/forgetfulness

13. Poor orientation to time and place
14. Dark circles under the eyes
15. Greyish tinge of skin
16. Poor work performance
17. Proneness to industrial/road accidents
18. Development of hypertension, heart diseases and even cancer
19. Poor growth in children
20. Proneness to infection and delayed healing.

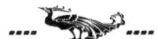

Chapter 2

Physiology of Sleep

What is Sleep?

Sleep is a state of subconsciousness, which occurs in the night or sometimes during the daytime and usually lasts for some hours. When conscious or awake, an individual is able to perform all activities like eating, drinking, learning, procreating etc. When asleep, an individual is not aware of the surroundings, does not move or respond to when spoken to or touched and is unable to perform routine activities.

Coma: A Prolonged Sleep

Coma is a prolonged state of deep sleep due to some disease or injury to the brain. In this state, the individual cannot be aroused or awakened even by strong stimuli unlike in sleep. Oxygen consumption by the brain is reduced in coma unlike in normal sleep where there is no change.

Other Sleep Like Unconsciousness

1. *Syncope* or *fainting* is a temporary loss of consciousness due to some abnormal changes in the body.
2. *Stupor* is a state of reduced or suspended consciousness, caused due to the shock, daze, intoxicants etc.
3. Brain death is said to occur when the regulatory mechanisms of the body controlling blood pressure,

respiration etc. collapse due to some injury to the brain or reduced blood supply to the brain. Brain death is said to occur when such a state lasts for more than 6-12 hours and the EEG (electro-encephalograph) shows no recording of brain waves.

How Long Can You Sleep?

The duration of sleep varies according to the age. Newborn babies sleep for up to 16 hours daily with several short intervals of wakefulness. As the child grows up there is a gradual diminution in the duration of sleep, to 7-8 hours, in adulthood. This also depends to some extent on the amount of manual work performed. In old age, about 5-6 hours of sleep supplemented by short naps in the daytime is observed.

How is Sleep Induced?

In spite of immense research work, the exact mechanism by which sleep is induced has not been discovered. In different parts of the brain there are nerve fibres (neurons), which form a network called the **Ascending Reticular Activating System** (A.R.A.S.). It has been postulated that when these fibres are electrically activated or stimulated, the person enters the state of wakefulness. In the absence of stimulation of the A.R.A.S., it is believed that the person goes to sleep.

Besides the A.R.A.S., there are two sleep centres made of nerve fibres which are responsible for producing the Slow-Wave Sleep (S.W.S.) and Rapid-Eye Movement (R.E.M.) Sleep, respectively. The sleep centre for S.W.S. is located in the medulla of the brain and uses a chemical substance called serotonin as the neurotransmitter for inducing S.W.S.

The R.E.M. sleep centre is located in "pons"—a part of the brain—and uses neuropinephrine as the neuro-transmitter for inducing R.E.M. sleep.

The Sleeping State

In a typical night of sleep, an adult enters two types of states, *i.e.* Slow-Wave Sleep (S.W.S.) or Non-Rapid Eye-

Movement Sleep (N.R.E.M.) and Fast-Wave Sleep (F.W.S.) or Rapid-Eye Movement (R.E.M.) sleep.

Initially, the person enters into the state of S.W.S., which progresses in an orderly way in four stages from light to deep sleep. Thus, there is a progressive reduction in consciousness and an increasing resistance to being awakened. During this state of sleep the muscles are relaxed, heart and respiratory rates decreased and the metabolic activity slows down.

In the state of fast-wave sleep, there are rapid eye movements, due to which it is called R.E.M. sleep. This stage is reached after about 90 minutes from the start of the

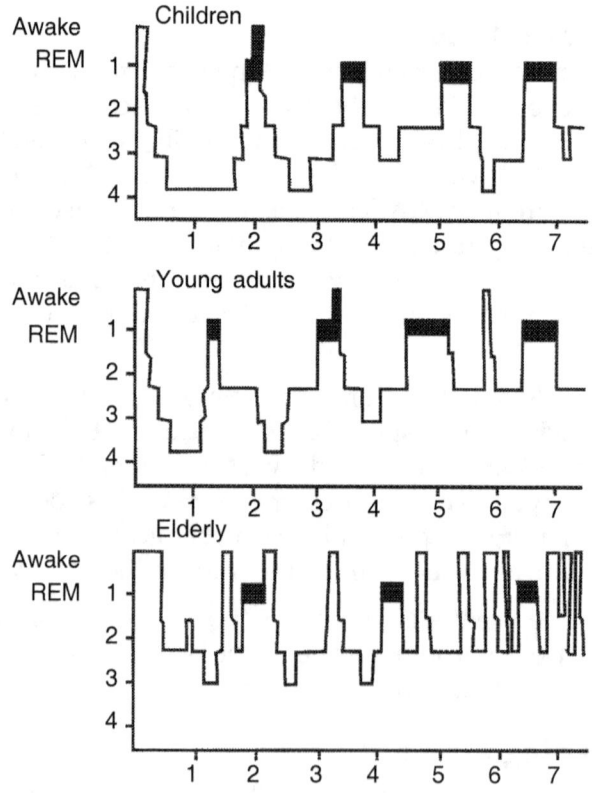

Fig. 1: Normal sleep cycle at various ages

sleep cycle. This stage of sleep is also associated with dreaming. During the R.E.M. sleep, the middle ear muscles are active, penile erection occurs, heartbeat and respiration becomes irregular and there are occasional twitching of the muscles of the limb. Since muscle tone is very much reduced during R.E.M. sleep, the muscle twitching do not produce any injury or awaken the individual. Teeth grinding may also occur in some individuals.

There are 4-6 R.E.M periods per night and it constitutes about 25 per cent of total sleep time. Thus, the sleep cycle consisting of R.E.M. and N.R.E.M. phases repeats itself about 5 times during the night. After the second cycle, the interval between periods of R.E.M. sleep becomes longer. Also, as the morning approaches, an individual spends less time in the deeper stages of S.W.S. and awakens periodically.

Does Sleep Change Our Physiology?

Yes! Certain changes in the body systems are observed during the sleep.

1. Nervous system

A state of drowsiness lasting for a few minutes usually precedes sleep. Different sensations are diminished starting from the sense of smell. A sleeping person can be easily disturbed without an attempt by him to correct his position or prevent a fall from the cot. Muscle tone is reduced—all the muscles get relaxed during sleep. Exciting dreams may occur associated with a powerful penile erection and ejaculation (wet dreams). Characteristic EEG changes are recorded during different stages of sleep.

2. Cardiovascular system

The heartbeat rate is reduced by as much as 10-30 beats per minute. During the first 3-4 hours, the blood pressure falls by 10-30 mm Hg and later, slowly rises until waking up. When exciting dreams occur, the blood pressure may increase during this period.

3. Respiratory system

During sleep the respiratory rate as well as depth of respiration is slowed down. In some individuals, breathing can stop temporarily, giving rise to a condition called sleep-apnea. In R.E.M. sleep respiration may become irregular in pattern.

4. Urinary (excretory) system

During sleep the output of urine is diminished as also the concentration of it. Due to accumulation of urine during sleep, bacterial multiplication may occur speedily. Sweat secretion is increased during sleep.

5. Digestive system

The digestive system is as active as during the period of wakefulness. There is a marginal decrease in the metabolic rate during sleep.

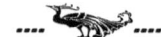

— Chapter 3 —

How to Have Sound Sleep

There are certain factors that are helpful in producing a sound sleep. These are dependent on the environment inside the bedroom, the surrounding areas and on factors pertaining to the personality and health of the individual.

1. Ventilation in the Bedroom

The bedroom should be ideally located in that part of the house which has good access to air and sunlight. No air-conditioner, cooler or fan can substitute the natural and fresh air flowing through windows and doors of our house. Cross-ventilation is an added advantage giving rise to good supply of air in the house.

Sunlight should be allowed to enter the bedroom during the day since the ultraviolet rays are very beneficial for maintaining the internal ambience of the whole house, including the bedroom. The humidity is reduced, various invisible micro-organisms are destroyed and the sleeping person gets a free dose of Vitamin D and energy for the whole day.

2. Temperature of the Bedroom

The normal room temperature accepted internationally is 30ºC (86ºF) for attaining a sound sleep and maintenance of the "sleep-awake" cycle. Therefore, for sleeping comfortably it is very important to maintain this temperature in the bedroom. In winters, room-heaters may be used to raise the room temperature. Similarly, in summer air-conditioners can reduce the summer heat.

3. Lighting in the Bedroom

The lighting arrangement in the bedroom should be such that it is soothing to the eyes and the mind. It is advisable to use fluorescent table lights rather than filament bulbs in the bedroom. Fluorescent lights emit less heat than filament bulbs and are cool and simulate natural light. These lights should be preferably switched off before going to sleep, otherwise a zero watt bulb, preferably a blue colour one, may be left on for the night.

4. Wall-painting in the Bedroom

The walls of the bedroom should preferably be painted with a blue, violet, indigo or green distemper. These colours are very soothing both for the nerves and the mind. Dark colours cause depression, whereas red and associated hues give rise to frequent quarrels among the family members.

5. Electronic Gadgets

No electronic gadget like television, music system or computer should be kept in the bedroom. This is because the electromagnetic radiations adversely affect the mind and the sleep patterns.

6. Photographs, Wall-hangings, Wallpapers, Showpieces

Ideally no photograph, wall-hanging or showpiece should be kept in the bedroom. A family photograph can help in binding the family together and maintaining unity, integrity and peace in the family. Pregnant women can have photographs of smiling babies which can induce sound sleep during their pregnancy and a painless delivery. Those with a taste for wall-hangings, wallpapers and decoratives should select those, which have a soothing effect on their mind. Wall-clocks in the room should not have luminous dials or chimes, because these can disturb the sleep at night due to their light and sound.

7. Dressing Table
The dressing table in the bedroom should not be kept in such a way that the image of the occupant is reflected on waking up.

8. Bed-mattresses, Pillows, etc.
The bed is the most important object of the bedroom that determines the sleep quality of the occupants. The length of the bed should be adequate since our body lengthens by a few inches when we lie down. This is more relevant for individuals with a height more than 6 feet since standard bed size is 6'x6'. If the legs of the person hang beyond the foot end, he will not wake up refreshed in the morning. Sleeping on "charpoys" or "folding beds" can also give rise to backache and poor sleep since the backbone does not get enough support during the night.

Mattresses should be firm and preferably made of coir and foam, which can be used according to the weather conditions. Mattresses made up of foam alone or an uneven mattress can give rise to backache.

Ideally, pillows should not be used. This is because the pillows tend to bend the neck forward causing abnormal curvature of cervical spine and even lead to Cervical Spondylosis in individuals with short necks. A contour pillow, which supports the head and neck properly, may be used if required. A wedge-shaped pillow below the knees is also a good alternative for relaxing the backbone.

Pregnant women can slip an extra pillow under the belly for support.

Bedsheets and blankets should be soft, comfortable to use and clean. If their colours are blue, violet, indigo or green, they exert a soothing effect on the mind.

9. Pests

Certain pests in the bedroom like mosquitoes, houseflies, cockroaches, ants, bedbugs can disturb the sleep of the occupants. These pests should be destroyed by regular usage of insecticides, especially the spray-type repellants, mosquito-nets and other devices. Sunlight should be allowed to enter the bedroom during the daytime by opening all doors, and windows to the extent possible and safe. This can prevent humidity and destroy many of these pests. An exhaust fan or an A.C. can also remove the pests, bad odour and humidity in the bedroom.

10. Noise Pollution

It is very difficult to sleep if there is noise from the loudspeakers, music systems, televisions, people's quarrelling, playing children etc.

This type of noise pollution in the adjoining rooms or neighbourhood should be minimised in order to attain a sound sleep.

11. Regular and Timely Sleeping Habits

Due to the "biological-clock" in our body, a regular "sleep-awake" cycle is maintained. Therefore, sleeping regularly at a fixed time helps us to wake up fresh daily. Irregular sleep timings can give rise to sleep disorders and their associated symptoms.

12. Daytime Activities

People, who are physically active throughout the day, rarely find problem in attaining sleep. A labourer, a farmer or a rickshaw-puller is rarely known to suffer from sleep problem. They are known to sleep like "a log of wood" due to their physical activity. In contrast, people with sedentary lifestyle are known to suffer from sleep disorders. Also people, who have the habit of sleeping for long hours in the afternoon, rarely get a good sleep at night. Thus, physical activity or early-morning exercise is a must for attaining good sleep at night.

13. Music, Mantras, Meditation and Reading

A light music, devotional songs, a lullaby or recitation of Gayatri Mantra or Om or any other *japa* or prayer can be very beneficial for getting a good sleep. Meditation, Reiki, Pranayama, Shavasana etc. can also soothe mind and body. Reading of a religious book just before sleep is also useful.

14. Positive Attitude Towards Life

People with a positive attitude towards life rarely yield to stress and tensions, which are the main culprits for sleep disorders. Hence, this approach is beneficial.

15. Other Factors

Research has proved that sexual intercourse before sleep or even fore-play can prove to be more powerful than sleeping pills. **Vaastu Shastra** recommends that the location of the bedroom should be ideally in the south-west or the position of the head should be in that direction. The best position for sleeping is lying on the back or "Shavasana" posture. Yoga recommends lying down on the right side since while lying on the right side, the left nostril produces a evolving effect on the body and mind. This produces a night of undisturbed sleep and is called "Baba Shaiya" and "Simha Shaiya."

A hot water bath or oil massage is very useful as is the burning of incense or aromatic oils.

Recommendations for sound sleep

1. A well-ventilated, sun-facing bedroom
2. Cosy bedroom with comfortable temperature
3. Soft lighted bedroom

4. Walls of the bedroom painted blue, violet, indigo or green
5. Minimum electronic gadgets in the bedroom
6. A family photograph in the bedroom
7. Wall-clocks without luminous dials or chimes
8. A normal size bed with a coir-foam mattress, contour pillows, clean bedsheets and blankets of compatible colour.
9. Pests removed by regular spraying of insecticides
10. Sound-proof room with no noise pollution in the surrouding area
11. Regular and timely sleeping habits
12. Regular physical activity. No daytime naps
13. A light, non-spicy, non-oily dinner about 2 to 3 hours before sleep
14. A cup of hot milk before dinner
15. Music, mantras, meditation and reading religious books are useful
16. Positive attitude towards life is beneficial
17. Other factors: sex, location of bedroom in south-west, sleeping posture, hot water bath or oil massage.

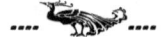

Chapter 4

Sleep Disorders

Sleep disorders are caused by factors mostly related to our lifestyle, environment, dietary habits and health problems.

1. Lifestyle

1. Stress and tension

Stress and tension constitute an integral part of the modern civilization. Even the children are not spared. The strain of modern life takes its toll on the mental peace and sleeping habits of the people. Keeping up with hectic office schedules, deadlines of assignments, preparation for exams and co-ordinating with the household chores lead to improper and inadequate sleep patterns among individuals.

2. Erratic lifestyle

Certain people have very erratic and irregular lifestyle. They do not follow a fixed time for eating, sleeping or in their regular activities. Due to their variable sleep timings, the sleep-awake cycle is not maintained leading to inadequate or poor quality of sleep. This is also seen in people going to late night parties, movies or discotheques.

3. Shift-duty

Persons on shift duties like the policemen, medical practitioners and factory workers have a uncertain sleep timings. Sometimes they sleep during the day and at other times at night. This disturbs the circadian rhythm and undermines sleep.

4. Daytime sleeping
People who are in the habit of sleeping in the morning or afternoon, especially the elderly individuals, unemployed or anti-social elements, rarely get a good sleep at night. This is because they have already met their requirement of sleep for the night.

5. Physical activity
People who lead a sedentary lifestyle without much physical activity, rarely get a good sleep. In contrast people who are involved in physical activities rarely have problems with sleep.

6. Mental problems
The mental problems which affect sleep are loss of job, divorce, accident, death of a beloved, rape, suicide attempt, murder, hijacking/kidnapping, loss in business etc. These can cause either temporary or long-term sleep disorders.

7. Regular intake of stimulating/ intoxicating substances
People who regularly consume alcohol, tea, coffee, drugs, tobacco (cigarette, "zarda", "gutka", "khaini") have problems in their sleep. These contain nicotine, a substance which stimulates the brain and in fact prevents the person from sleep. Soft drinks and chocolates contain caffeine that is also a stimulant and keeps the mind alert. Sudden stoppage of these substances can also disturb sleep due to withdrawal symptoms.

8. Irregular bowel habits
People, who are unable to evacuate their bowels regularly, are also prone to develop sleep disorders. This is because when the waste products of digestion remain in the bowel for long, certain toxic chemicals are produced. These

substances affect the sleep cycle both in the quality and quantity of sleep.

9. Viewing or reading violent, pornographic, exciting, horror movies/books

In modern society, cable television has become popular among people of all ages. Sex, violence, horror and adventure are depicted in almost all programmes. People, who watch such movies/programmes just before sleep, find such scenes haunting them during sleep cycle, which results in disturbed sleep.

Similarly, people, who are in the habit of reading books containing similar material just before sleep, rarely attain sound sleep.

2. Environmental Factors

1. Poor ventilation

Nobody can deny that the sleep attained under the shade of a tree where there is both air and sunlight, is highly blissful and cannot be substituted by anything. But people, who have restricted or no access to natural air and sunlight in their bedroom, don't always get a good sleep. Lack of air and sunlight can increase the humidity of the room, hasten growth of micro-organisms and pests, and deprive the body of free supply of Vitamin D and pure oxygen.

2. Extreme room temperature

If the temperature in the bedroom is very high in summer or very cold in winter, the occupants have problems in attaining a sound sleep. This can be improved by using coolers, air-conditioners, fans etc. during the summer and room-heaters/flowers in winter. Very cold or damp atmosphere in the bedroom is also not conducive for sleep.

3. Lighting in the room

The lighting in the bedroom should be arranged in such a way that it gets maximum sunlight during the daytime.

Therefore, the curtains should be removed and the windows opened during the daytime and the windows closed and curtains drawn during the evening and night. There should be soft fluorescent lights in the bedroom preferably of low wattage and zero watt bulbs preferably of blue, green or violet colours.

4. Bed and accessories

To sleep comfortably, people should use hard-bed instead of "charpoys" or "folding-beds", which can give rise to backache and disturbed sleep. People of height above 6 feet on undersized beds (less than 6 feet) do not get a sound sleep, because their legs tend to hang down from the foot end of the bed. Colour therapy experts have observed that people who use red, yellow or orange blankets, bedsheets and pillow-covers, get disturbed sleep with nightmares. In contrast, blue, green, indigo and violet colours are very soothing to the mind and body. According to Vaastu Shastra, people who sleep with their heads in the North direction, spend sleepless nights with lots of dreams and even nightmares.

5. Pests

Mosquitoes, houseflies, cockroaches, ants and bedbugs can disturb the sleep of the occupants of the bedroom. They are commonly seen in bedrooms, which are not cleaned regularly or where humidity is high.

6. Other factors in the bedroom

Certain factors relevant to Vaastu Shastra and Feng Shui also affect the sleep. Electronic gadgets in the bedroom like the television, VCR, music system etc., affect the body and mind. Photographs of dead people, naked photos or frightening pictures also adversely affect the sleep pattern. If the location of the dressing table is such that the reflection of the person falls on it on waking up, it is not good for sleep either. The walls of the bedroom should be ideally painted blue, green, indigo or violet in order to soothe the nervous system and get a sound sleep. Overcrowding in the bedroom, or using the bedroom as a kitchen or drawing room or for doing office-work or studying hampers sleep.

2. Noise Pollution

Excessive noise in the bedroom or adjoining rooms or in the neighbourhood can disturb the sleep. The noise pollution can be from TVs, music systems, children playing, quarrels, marriages or *jagrans* using loudspeakers or an orchestra or chiming clocks etc.

3. Dietary Factors

A heavy meal just before sleep is best avoided.

People, who eat fast foods or junk foods like chowmein, burgers, spicy dishes or non-vegetarian food at dinner, may not get a sound sleep. All these contain excessive fat content, which takes a long time in digestion. Lack of fibre can also give rise to constipation, which is another cause of insomnia.

4. Medical Problems

Indiscriminate use of medicines, including sedatives (which calm the mind) and hypnotics (which induce sleep), can disturb the sleep pattern. This can be in the form of tolerance (requiring higher doses for producing effect), habituation, worsening of sleep or abrupt discontinuation or changeover to newer medication.

Certain medicines are known to disturb sleep. These are appetite suppressants, anti-allergens, corticosteroids, thyroid hormones, androgens, excess Vitamin A and medicines for controlling vomiting, cough, asthma, hypertension, depression, Parkinsonism, peptic ulcer and body swelling.

Certain physical ailments affecting the body can disturb sleep. Pain due to arthritis, angina, backache, accidents, headache, fever, operations, delivery, peptic ulcer, abdominal or renal colic etc. can disturb the sleep pattern. Other diseases, which affect sleep, are asthma, increased urination (due to diabetes, kidney diseases, enlarged prostate), itching (due to skin disease), heart diseases (chest pain, breathing problem or high blood pressure), overactive thyroid (with increased heartbeat, sweating), worms, mental indigestion, illnesses, epilepsy, brain tumour. Constipation is also a major cause of sleep disorders.

5. Other Causes

The problem of sleeplessness may be a part of familial (genetic) disorders. It has been observed that if parents or grandparents suffer from insomnia, the person is about 5 times more susceptible to this problem.

1. Nutrition Status is also an important factor for the initiation of sleep, since the body and mind are interconnected. Thus people with severe malnutrition as well as those with over nutrition or obesity suffer from sleep disorders.

2. Hormonal Changes in the body, especially in women may be responsible for lack of sleep. Most women don't get adequate sleep during menstrual period, pregnancy, after delivery and at menopause. Premenstrual tension in adolescent girls is another cause of sleep disturbance. When a person travels abroad by plane, he develops certain symptoms due to the travel through several time zones. These are collectively known as "jet lag". These symptoms are our inability to sleep at night, daytime fatigue, poor concentration, headache, poor appetite and constipation.

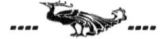

Chapter 5

Snoring

Like other sounds, snoring is caused by vibrations that make the particles in the air to form sound waves. When we speak, our vocal cords vibrate to form our voice. While our stomach growls, our stomach and intestines vibrate when air and food move through them. During sleep the turbulent air flow causes the tissues of the nose and throat to vibrate giving rise to snoring.

Sleep apnea, a sleep disorder characterised by snoring as well as any kind of interrupted sleep causes mental decline. It has already been associated with high blood pressure heart diseases and diabetes. Each pause in breathing called apnea lasts from a few seconds to minutes and may occur five to thirty times or even more per hour. Frequent interruptions of sleep affects memory and other brain functions.

How common is Snoring?

Study shows that 45 per cent of men and 30 per cent women snore on a regular basis. Those people who do not snore may snore after a viral illness, consumption of alcohol or taking some medications. We normally think of heavy built with a thick neck as a snorer while a thin woman with a small neck can snore just as loudly. Snoring is aggravated by excess weight and may get worse with age.

Causes of Snoring

Air flows from our nose or mouth to our lungs when we breath. At the time of exercising, air moves faster and produces sounds rapidly as we breath. Since air is moving in and out of the nose as well as mouth more quickly it causes more turbulence in the airflow causing sharpen vibration of the tissues in nose and mouth. While we are sleeping a certain areas at the back of throat sometimes narrows. Some amount of air passing through this smaller opening causes the tissues surrounding the opening to vibrate and that in turn results in the production of the sound called snoring.

Mouth Breathing and Snoring

It is ideal to breath through the nose. It acts as a humidifier, heater and filter for the incoming air. Some people can not breath through their nose due to some kind of blockage of the nasal passage. This can also be caused due to deviation of the nasal septum, allergies, infections, swelling of turbinates or tonsils in the back of the throat. In adults common causes of nasal obstruction are septa deviations from a broken nose or allergies while in children, tonsils in the back of the throat are often causes of the obstruction necessitating breathing through their mouth. Most of the mouth breathers snore as the flow of air through mouth causes greater vibration of tissues.

The soft palate and snoring

The soft palate is a muscular extension of the bony roof of mouth separating the back of mouth from nasal passages. Shaped like a sheet attached at their sides hangs freely in the back of mouth has importance while breathing and swallowing. If the soft palate is too long or loose it causes vibration and in turn the snoring.

Narrowed airways and snoring

The tonsils are designed to detect and fight infections. It is observed that the tonsils sometimes do not return to their normal size after the infection is cured. Enlarged tonsil narrows the leading to faster vibration causing snoring. The uvula is suspended from the centre and back of the soft palate. If it is abnormally long or thick it can contribute to snoring. The tongue can narrow the space through which air flows in the pharynx leading to vibrations and snoring.

Stage of sleep and snoring

Sleep consists of several stages like R.E.M. rapid eye movement and non rapid eye movement. Snoring can occur in any stage but it is common in R.E.M. sleep due to loss of muscle tone characteristic at this stage of sleep when the brain sends the signal to all the muscles of the body to relax. The tongue palate and throat can collapse when they relax causing the airway to narrow and worsen snoring.

Sleeping position and snoring

Whenever we are sleeping or lying down, gravity acts to pull on the tissues of the body. When we lie on our back, gravity pulls the palate tonsils and tongue backwards. It often narrows the airway to cause turbulence in air flow, tissue vibration, and snoring.

How alcohol affects snoring?

The root cause of snoring is vibration of the tissues while breathing. Consumption of alcohol leads to enhanced relaxation of muscles during sleep. While the muscles of palate, tongue, neck and pharynx relax more, the airway collapses more. This leads to a narrower airway and greater tissue vibration and worsened snoring.

Evalution of snoring

To thoroughly evaluate someone with a snoring problem it would certainly be of importance to talk to the person's bed partner or family members. The history and physical examination to be considered covers sleep pattern, day time symptoms of sleepiness, daytime napping and frequency of awakening at night, body weight, neck circumference, besides throat, nasal as well as oral an examination to determine how narrow the oral and nasal passages are.

Treatments for snoring

Following are the non- surgical treatment of snoring:

1. Behavioural Changes

Such changes include weight loss changing sleeping positions, avoiding alcohol, giving up smoking and changing of medications that may be the cause of snoring. Losing weight improves snoring. Snoring is worse while lying flat on the back. To help this problem make a pocket into the back of snorer's pajama top. A tennis or any small ball in this pocket would frequently force the snorer to roll over during sleep on his/her side.

2. Dental devices

Snoring is exacerbated by normal air flow through a narrowed passage in the throat. This narrowing is partly caused by the tongue and palate falling back. The dental devices have been developed which hold the jaw forward and improve the snoring in 70 to 90% cases. These devices are recommended for the individuals with primary snoring and also did not benefit or could not qualify for the above behavioural changes. Dental devices are best made by dentist to ensure correct fit without causing any sort of problem.

3. Nasal devices and medications

The snoring can be alleviated with some nasal devices or medications for those people who have narrow nasal passage. The anterior nasal valve which is in the front part of the nose is opened by breath-rite strips. These strips improve snoring if this is the main or only area of narrowing. Nasal sprays help if the nasal mucosal swelling from allergies or the irritation causes the problem. These measures are helpful to people who snore if they have the upper respiratory infections causing swelling of the airway passages.

4. Nasal CPAP

It is a device to produce continues positive airway pressure commonly used for patients with a clinical diagnosis of obstructive sleep apnea. This device reduces the snoring and other symptoms of obstructive sleep apnea. Air pressure is adjusted for each patient depending on the parameters of a sleep study. The drawback of this CPAP device is that it is bulky, noisy and uncomfortable for patients to wear throughout the night.

Highlights of snoring

- ❑ Vibrating tissues in the airways of the nose and throat cause snoring
- ❑ Turbulent airflow through narrowed airways cause vibrations resulting in snoring
- ❑ Stage of sleep, sleeping position use of medications and consumption of alcohol is responsible for snoring
- ❑ Snoring is the problem for the bed partner of the snorer and other family members
- ❑ Snoring in some cases is a sign of other problems
- ❑ There are surgical as well as non surgical treatment for snoring.

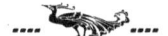

Chapter 6

Nightmares

Nightmares are bad dreams that cause horror, terror or fear. Normally the content of nightmares revolves around imminent harm being caused to the individual who is being chased threatened or injured etc. The nightmares also involve the previous threatening or horrifying circumstances that had been part of any traumatic event.

People might experience frightening dreams about terrorists, aeroplane crashes, collapsing buildings, fire and people jumping from buildings etc. A rape survivor naturally gets disturbing dreams about the rape itself or in some cases the experience was frightening being held at knife point. The nightmares can occur multiple times during a night. The individuals see the same dream repeatedly or sometimes they experience different dreams with a similar theme. The individuals when awaken from nightmares report feelings of fear and anxiety. Nightmares occur mostly during rapid eye movement (REM) sleep which occurs on and off throughout the night. REM sleep periods become longer with the result the dreaming tends to be more intense in the second half of night.

How common are nightmares

The prevalence of nightmares varies by age group and their gender. These are first experienced between the ages of three and six years. 10 to 15 per cent of children during this age has nightmares which are severe enough to cause anxiety in their parents. It does not mean that children with nightmares have a psychological disorder. The children who develop nightmares in the absence of traumatic events typically grow out of them with age.

Every second adult reports at least an occasional nightmare. It is seen that 7 to 8 per cent of the adult population suffer from the chronic nightmares. Women report nightmares more often than men do.

Psychological treatment for nightmares

The clients are taught basic strategies that may help them get quality sleep. The treatment involves helping the clients change the endings of their nightmares while they are awake so that the ending is no larger upsetting. Psychologists use the behavioural techniques as the treatment of nightmares for crime victims and the sexual assault survivors.

What happens if nightmares are left untreated?

Nightmares can be a chronic mental health problem for some individuals. It is not clear why they plague some people and not others. Nightmares are common in the early phases after a traumatic experience and gradually reduce in intensity with time without treatment. It takes about three months to subside substantially. If the symptoms persist then a mental health professional can be consulted. The nightmares should in any case be treated in time otherwise it would become chronic. It would continue to harm the person throughout the life. One should try to forget the horrible incidents of past.

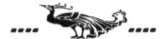

Chapter 7

Sleepwalking

Sleepwalking is a disorder characterised by walking or any other activities while seemingly still asleep. Occasionally non-sensical talking occurs with person's eyes commonly open looking right at you. This activity occurs during middle childhood and adolescence. About 15 per cent of children between 4-12 years of age experience sleepwalking. Persons with certain inherited genes have greater tendency towards sleepwalking. An average sleepwalker experiences four to five complete sleep cycles per night. Sleepwalker has no memory of his or her behaviour upon walking.

The sleepwalking activity may also include simply sitting up, appearing awake while actually asleep, getting up and walking around besides complex activities such as moving furniture, going to the bathroom, dressing and undressing etc. Some people even drive a car while being actually asleep.

A person sleep walking should not be awakened and it is a misconception and the other misconception is that a person cannot be injured when sleep walking. Injuries caused by such events for sleepwalkers are common as tripping and loss of balance.

Common symptoms of sleepwalking

1. Quietly walking around the room; often running with attempt to escape.
2. On questioning the person sleepwalking fails to answer accurately.

3. Some children while sleepwalking repeatedly show certain behaviours.

Treatment for sleepwalking
1. Getting adequate sleep
2. Meditating or doing relaxation exercises
3. Keep safe sleeping environment
4. Lock the doors and windows
5. Sleep on the ground to prevent falling
6. Remove obstacles in the room
7. Place an alarm or bell on the bedroom door
8. Read some spiritual literature before sleeping.

Medical treatment for sleepwalking is necessary if there is the possibility of injury, continued behaviour is causing significant family disruption or other measures have proven inadequate.

Prevention of sleepwalking
1. Avoid use of alcohol or central nervous system depressants.
2. Avoid overwork resulting in fatigue.
3. Avoid or minimize stress anxiety and conflict which does worsen the condition.

Highlights of sleepwalking
- ❑ It is not a serious disorder but the children can be injured by object during sleep walking
- ❑ Prolonged disturbed sleep may be associated with school and behavioural issues
- ❑ Although it is frightening and disruptive over the short term, sleep walking is not associated with any long term complications
- ❑ Sleepwalking is fully curable.

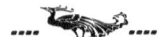

Chapter 8

Sleepiness

At times everyone feels sleepy. Sleepiness interferes with daily routine and activities reducing the ability to function properly. A person may not feel sleepy while talking or listening to music at a party but can fall asleep while driving home afterward.

Following are the symptoms of sleepiness.

1. Not getting enough sleep regularly
2. Getting poor quality asleep
3. Falling asleep when driving
4. Struggle to stay awake while watching television or reading
5. Lack of concentration at work or home
6. Having difficulty in paying attention
7. Another telling you that you are sleepy
8. Loss of memory with difficulty in remembering
9. Having difficulty in controlling emotions
10. Taking naps frequently.

Causes of Sleepiness

Sleepiness can be due to many reasons such as body's natural daily sleep wake cycles, inadequate sleep, sleep disorders or certain drugs.

Nature has made sleep wake cycle. Daily there are two periods when our body experiences a natural tendency towards sleepiness generally during the late night from midnight to 7 a.m. and again between 1 p.m. and 4 p.m. If you are awake during these two timings, you have a higher risk of falling sleep unintentionally especially if you didn't get enough sleep.

Many people do not get enough time to sleep. Firstly evaluate their daily activities of sleep wake patterns to determine as to have much sleep they get. If you are sleeping for less than eight hours then more of sleep may be needed. You have to gradually increase your sleeping time. Move to bed 15 minutes earlier each night for about four to five nights. This way you can increase your time of sleep without causing a sudden change in schedule. Alternatively you can have nap daily for about an hour or so if the schedules do not permit early bedtime.

Medications do not help problems of sleepiness; rather make it worse. Caffeine reduces sleepiness and increases alertness but only temporarily. Similarly, alcohol induces sleep but can disrupt sleep later in the night. Medications are prescribed for patients in certain situations. Short term use of sleeping pills has been helpful for patients of acute insomnia while long term use of sleep medication is recommended only for specific sleep disorders.

If you are sleepy, avoid driving. Avoid driving between midnight and 7 a.m. In case you are a shift worker then use caffeine only during the first part of the shift to promote alertness at night. If you are getting enough sleep but even then you feel sleepy during the day, check with your medical consultant to be sure that your sleepiness is not due to a sleep disorder.

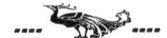

Chapter 9

Hypersomnia

Hypersomnia or so called as excessive sleepiness is a condition in which a person has the feeling of sleeping during the day. Such people can fall asleep at any time at work or even while driving.they also suffer from other sleep related problems which include lack of energy and trouble of not thinking clearly. As per the study conducted by National Sleep Foundation around 40 per cent of people have symptoms of hypersomnia from time to time.

Causes of Hypersomnia

There are several causes of hypersomnia such as day time sleepiness and interruptions of breathing during sleep, not getting enough sleep at night, overweight, drug or alcohol abuse, head injury or any neurological disease genetics having a relative with hypersomnia and many more.

Diagnosis of Hypersomnia

Consult your doctor if you feel drowsy during the day. The doctor should know your history regarding your sleeping habits that how much sleep you get at night and if you wake up at night then whether you fall asleep during the day. It will also be confirmed from you in case you are having any emotional problems or taking any medications interfering with your sleep.

Treatment of Hypersomnia

If you are suffering from hypersomnia, your doctor would prescribe the drugs including stimulants, antidepressants besides several medications such as Provigie and Xyrem. In case sleep apnea is diagnosed you are likely to be cured with treatment known as continuous positive airway pressure. Here you wear a mask over your nose while sleeping. The machine delivers a continuous flow of air into the nostrils is looked upto the mask. Air pressure flowing into the nostrils helps keep the airways open. If drowsiness persists during the day time because of some of medication you are taking then ask your doctor also who would change the medication to make you less sleepy. Try to go to bed early to get more sleep at night. Avoid alcohol or intoxicants of any kind.

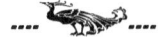

— Chapter 10 —

How to Tackle Sleep Disorders

Treatment of sleep disorders does not mean just popping in sleeping pills at night. It is multidisciplinary approach involving different modalities and systems of treatment for better and permanent results.

The treatment of sleep disorders is discussed under the following headings:

1. Changes in the Lifestyle
2. Dietary Management
3. Role of Physical Exercise in Treatment
4. Yoga and its Role in sleep Management
5. Naturopathy
6. Ayurvedic Remedies
7. Magnetotherapy
8. Acupressure and Reflexology
9. Chromotherapy
10. Music Therapy
11. Aromatherapy
12. Feng Shui
13. Medical Treatment—a Critical Analysis
14. Other General Tips

1. Changes in the Lifestyle

The lifestyle of an individual is one of the most important factors causing sleep disorder. Certain changes if brought about in the lifestyle of individuals with sleep disorder, can bring about long lasting positive results.

- ❑ People with a sedentary lifestyle can benefit remarkably by doing regular exercise and being active throughout the day.
- ❑ Stress can be overcome by practicing yoga, pranayam meditation, right attitude towards life and a positive approach.
- ❑ Minimise or give up completely the stimulants like tea, coffee, tobacco or alcohol.
- ❑ Irregular and late sleep-timings should also be avoided, visits to late night movies, parties and discotheques should be curtailed in order to enjoy the benefit of good sleep.
- ❑ Certain mental disorders like anxiety, depression, schizophrenia and other physical ailments affecting sleep should be appropriately treated.
- ❑ People who are in the habit of consuming sleeping pills regularly should stop doing so since its sedative effect wears off with regular usage.
- ❑ People with irregular bowel habits may sometimes develop sleep disorder. Therefore, they should make it a point to attend to nature's call every morning. A daytime sleeping can also affect the initiation of sleep.
- ❑ A short nap of less than an hour after a meal will do no harm to the sleeping pattern at night.
- ❑ No office work should be done at home especially in the bedroom at night.
- ❑ In times of stress, a prolonged foreplay or a sexual intercourse can help in getting sleep.

2. Dietary Management

Change faulty dietary habits to check sleep disorders. Certain do's and don'ts that you can follow:

3. Role of Physical Exercise

Physical exercise can directly or indirectly benefit people with sleep disorders. This is due to the following changes brought in the body:

Do's	Don'ts
1. Have dinner about 2 to 3 hours before going to sleep.	1. Do not go to sleep immediately after dinner.
2. Eat easily digestible food especially during dinner.	2. Do not eat food laced heavily with spices and fats.
3. Consume a well-balanced diet daily.	3. Avoid drinking tea, coffee, before going to sleep.
4. Have a fibre rich diet if suffering from constipation.	4. Do not smoke after dinner or before going to bed.
5. Eat lots of fruits, vegetables, sprouts and dal in the meals.	5. Do not skip the dinner.
6. Have three regular meals every day.	6. Do not drink alcohol before or with dinner.
7. Have a glass of warm milk after dinner as it contains serotonin, a sleep inducing agent.	7. Avoid vigorous dieting as it can give rise to sleeplessness.
	8. Soft drinks and chocolate should be avoided in excess since they contain caffeine.

1. Regular physical exercise releases the muscles tension in the body which is very conducive for initiation of sleep.
2. Physical or muscular relaxation is followed by mental relaxation because the body and the mind is

interlinked. The nervous system is thus smoothened for better sleep.
3. Exercise increases blood supply to different organs including the brain which gets a rich supply of oxygen for its nutrition.
4. Physical exercise tones up the gastrointestinal organs and increases digestion and absorption of food and prevents constipation. This prevents accumulation of toxic substances in the body.

Salient points to remember
- Exercise should be done at least 3 hours before sleep
- Vigorous exercise brings excessive fatigue which gives rise to problems in sleep initiation and maintenance of sleep
- A light stroll after dinner is very conducive in bringing sleep
- Light exercise of the neck and back is also very useful
- Exercise just before sleep increases the level of adrenaline which is more useful in keeping one awake rather than asleep
- A long walk or exercise in the morning is also very beneficial for attaining good sleep at night.

4. Yoga and its Role in Sleep Management
What is Yoga?
Yoga is an ancient Indian technique of integrating human personality at the physical, mental, moral and intellectual levels.

Maharishi Patanjali explained Yoga as *Chitta Vritti Nirodha* or control of the mind and body. He describes eight aspects (limbs) of Yoga which can be used to attain a healthy, happy and spiritual life. These are as follows:

1. "Yama" or moral principles like non-violence, truthfulness, honesty, celibacy and covetousness
2. "Niyama" or rules of discipline like purity, contentment, austerity, introspection and dedication to God
3. "Asanas" or yogic postures
4. "Pranayama" or control of breathing
5. "Pratyhara" or control of the mind or the sense organs
6. "Dharana" or concentration
7. "Dhyana" or meditation
8. "Samadhi" or a state of transcendental consciousness when the mind merges with the universal spirit.

Role of Yoga in the treatment of sleep disorders

(a) Yogasanas

Yogasanas refer to the yogic postures of the body which help with the physical, mental and spiritual development of the individual. Exercises can be classified according to the function they perform or their beneficial effect on the body.

Exercises that improve muscle strength

Weightlifting, barbell, dumbbell, clubs, springs (Bullworker), wrestling, push-ups, sit-ups.

Exercises that improve stamina

Brisk walking, skipping, running, cycling, swimming.

Exercises that promote special skills

Tennis, cricket, squash, badminton, table tennis, basketball, baseball, volleyball, football, rugby, hockey.

Exercises that maintain general fitness of the body

Aerobic exercises, dancing.

Exercises that improve muscle tone, strength, stamina, physical & mental function

Yogasana and Pranayama.

Differences between Physical Exercise and Yogasana

	Physical Exercise	**Yogasana**
1. Movement of body	Moves rapidly.	Moves slowly and uniformly.
2. Age Groups	Intensity varies as per age	Can be practiced by male, female and elderly.
3. Good effect on body	Strengthens the muscle.	Strengthens the mind and also the muscles.
4. Outcome	Causes anxiety, exhaustion & weariness.	Tones up the nervous and internal organs of body. Exhaustion & weariness not felt.
5. Development of body and mind	Mainly assists in development of body.	Developes body, mind & *prana*.
6. Flexibility of body	Lesser	More
7. Discontinuation	Cannot be given up suddenly.	Can be discontinued at any time.
8. Diet	High energy food is required.	Simple and pure food.
9. Prevention & cure of disease	Prevention possible.	Has curable powers.

Yogasanas Useful for Treatment of Sleep Disorders

For the sake of convenience these asanas may be divided into 4 groups.

1. Those done in the Supine Position—Shavasana-Matsyasana, Sarvangasana, Chakrasana.
2. Those done in the Prone Position—Dhanurasana, Makarasana.
3. Those done in the Sitting Position—Shasankasana, Paschimottanasana, Parvatasana.
4. Those done in the Standing Position—Shirshasana.

1. Supine Position

Shavasana (Corpse Pose) or relaxation pose (Mritasana)

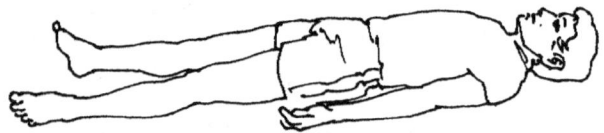

Fig. 4: Shavasana

Technique

- Lie flat in the supine position with feet about 1 foot apart, hands about 6" away from the body, palms facing upwards.
- Keep the eyes closed.
- Do not move any part of the body.
- Relax each part of the body starting from the legs upwards to the head.
- Keep the mind free from any thoughts.
- Breathe slowly and effortlessly.
- Concentrate on the breathing.

- Lie in this position for at least 10-15 minutes.

Precautions

- One must not fall off to sleep during this asana.
- Obese people with short neck require a small pillow or support at the back of the neck.

Matsyasana (Fish Pose)

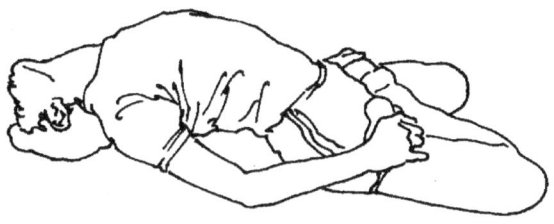

Fig. 5: Matsyasana

This asana is called Matsyasana because it is said that yogis could float on water like fishes in this asana by holding their breath.

Technique

- Assume a sitting position with the legs bent at the knees and the feet kept on opposite hip joints. The heels are adjusted in such a way that each presses the adjacent portion of the abdomen. This forms a foot-lock as in Padmasana.
- Bend backwards with the head resting on the crown and the weight of the body on the elbows.
- Push the neck backward and slightly raise the hip and chest upwards thus making an arch of the spine.
- Hold the toes on the corresponding side by hooking the fingers.
- Breathe deeply and stay in this position as long as possible.
- Then release the neck and let the head rest on the floor. Straighten the legs and relax the hands, elbows and the whole body.

- Repeat the asana, with the legs crossed the other way.

Precautions

The arching of the spine should be done slowly to avoid injury to spine.

Sarvangasana (Shoulder Stand)

It is a core exercise for all practitioners of Yoga and is sometimes called as "the mother of all asanas."

Technique

- Lie down in a supine position with legs and arms straight, feet together and palms facing downwards.
- Take a deep breath and lift both the legs slowly upwards till they are at right angle to the body.
- After exhaling pause for a few seconds.
- Inhale and lift legs, buttocks and lower back with the forearms so that the chin presses into the breastbone. Thus the entire weight of the body rests on the head, neck and shoulders and the arms are used for balancing.
- Focus the eyes on the big toes with the chin pressed against the chest and breathe slowly.
- Maintain this posture for 2-3 minutes.
- Exhale and bring down the legs after releasing the hands and the palms.

Precautions

- This asana should not be practiced by individuals with

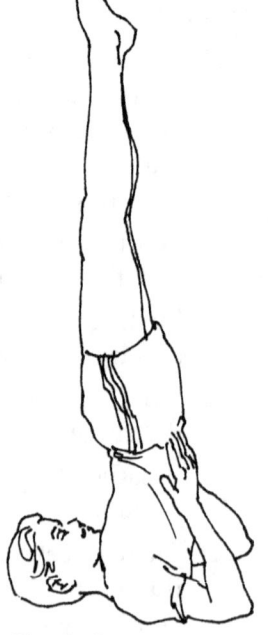

Fig. 6: Sarvangasana

high blood pressure, heart disease, cervical spondylitis and slipped disc.
- ❏ Obese individuals, people with weak backbone or abdominal muscles and beginners are advised to support their legs against a wall initially.
- ❏ It should be avoided during menstruation and advanced pregnancy.

Chakrasana (Wheel Pose)

Technique

- ❏ Lie on the back with the knees bent and feet about 12 inches apart flatly placed close to the buttocks.
- ❏ The arms are bent backward with palms under the shoulder region and fingers pointing towards the feet.
- ❏ Inhale and slowly raise the whole body upwards, resting on feet and palms.
- ❏ The head hangs downwards between the two stretched arms.

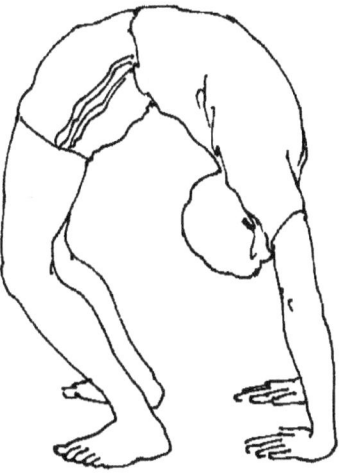

Fig. 7: Chakrasana

- ❏ Retain the position for 10-15 seconds and gradually increase the duration while continuing with normal breathing.
- ❏ Slowly come back to the original position while exhaling and rest in Shavasana for a few minutes.
- ❏ Practice up to three rounds.

Precautions

- ❏ Patients suffering from a slipped disc, ulcer, hernia, hypertension and heart diseases should avoid this asana. It is contraindicated during pregnancy.

2. Prone Position

Dhanurasana (Bow Pose)

Technique

- ❑ Lie down in the prone position (on the stomach) with the face and forehead touching the ground with the legs straight and the arms by the side.
- ❑ Exhale and bend the legs at the knee and hold them firmly by the hands at the ankles on the same side.
- ❑ Inhale, raise the thighs, chest and head simultaneously.
- ❑ The weight of the body should be on the navel and the head should be raised as high as possible with eyes looking upwards.
- ❑ This posture should be held as long as it is felt comfortable.
- ❑ Some authors recommend mild rocking movement on the abdomen, which bears the weight.
- ❑ Repeat this three to five times.

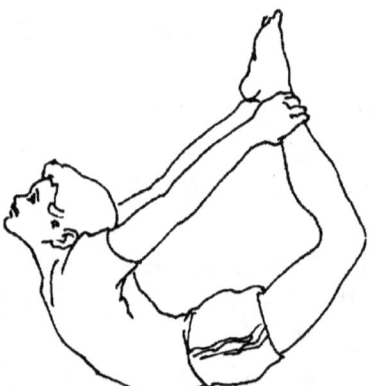

Fig. 8: Dhanurasana

Precautions

- ❑ This asana should not be done by those suffering from high blood pressure, slipped disc, hernia, colitis, duodenal and heart diseases.

Makarasana (Crocodile Pose)

Technique

- Lie flat on the stomach with the legs fully stretched and straight.
- Raise the head and shoulders.
- Fold the hands, place the elbows on the floor and hold the face and chin in the palms.
- Keep the elbows in such a way that there is no excess pressure on the neck or back.
- Relax the whole body and close the eyes breathing normally.
- It should be done for as long as possible.

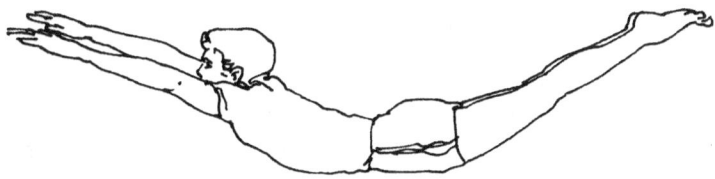

Fig. 9: Makarasana

- A variation is to place the palm on opposite shoulder and rest them with the face on the crossed hands.

Precautions

- Those who develop severe pain in the back or neck while doing this asana, should not practice it.

3. Sitting Position

Shasankasana (Hare Pose)

Technique

- Sit with legs folded backwards, heels apart, knees and toes together. (Vajrasana)

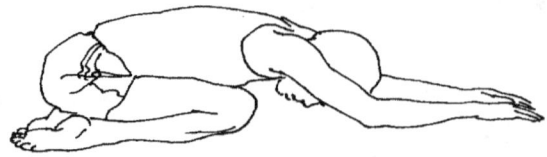

Fig. 10: Shasankasana

- Let both the hips fit in between the heels.
- Inhale and slowly raise the arms over the head.
- While exhaling, slowly bend forward, resting the palms on the floor and the abdomen pressing against the thighs.
- Bring the face downwards and touch the floor with the forehead without raising the buttocks.
- Inhale and come back to the original position.
- Repeat three to five times.

Precautions

- This exercise should not be done by persons suffering from cervical spondylitis, lumbar spondylitis, vertigo and hypertension.

Paschimottanasana (Back-stretching Pose)

Technique

- Sit on the floor with the legs outstretched, feet together and hands on the knees.
- Relaxing the whole body slowly bend forward from the hips, sliding the hands down the legs. Try to grasp the big toes with the fingers and thumbs. If not possible hold the heels, ankles or any part of the legs that can be reached comfortably.
- Hold this position for a few seconds.
- Keep the legs straight, bend the elbows and gently bring the trunk down towards the legs keeping a firm grip on the toes, feet or legs. Touch the knees with the forehead and hold in this position for as long as comfortable.

- Slowly return to the original position.
- Relax and repeat the exercise two to three times.

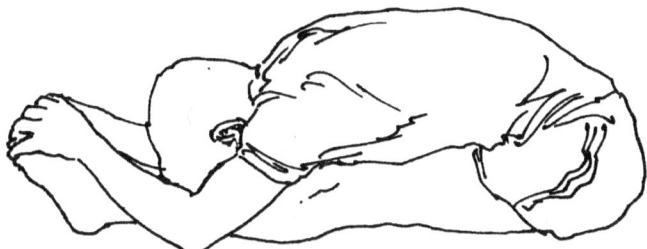

Fig. 11: Paschimottanasana

Precautions

- People who suffer from a slipped disc, lumbar spondylitis or sciatica should not perform this asana.
- Similarly those with cardiac problems, hernia and those who have undergone abdominal surgery should avoid this asana.

Parvatasana (Mountain Pose)

Technique

- Sit either in Vajrasana or padmasana keeping the spine and neck straight.
- Fold the hands with palm touching each other as in namaskara mudra.
- Close the eyes and inhaling, raise both the hands above the head.
- Allow the hands to stretch to the maximum. Look straight and remain in this position for some time, breathing slowly and deeply.
- Return to the normal position while exhaling.
- Repeat 10 to 15 times.

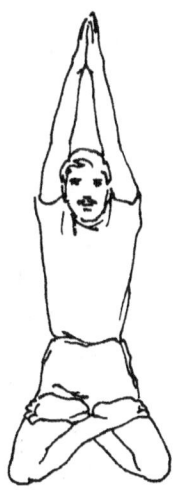

Fig. 12: Parvatasana

4. Standing Position

Shirshasana (Headstand Pose)

Technique

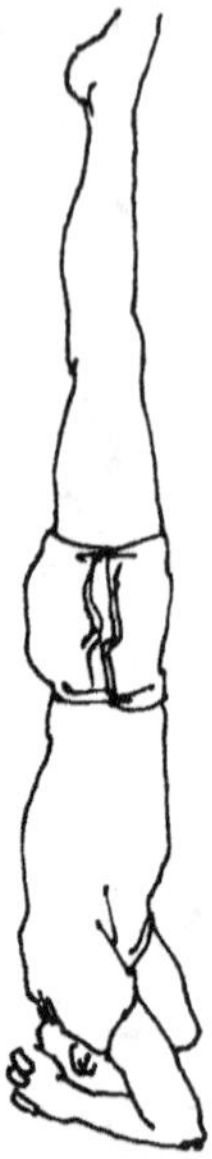

- Spread a blanket and kneel down on elbows and knees. The elbows are placed in the line of the shoulder joints.
- The fingers are fully interlocked and the two palms joined together.
- The crown of the head is placed on the blanket with the locked palms touching the back of the head.
- Move the knees closer to the face and slowly raise the legs initially by bending the knees and bearing some weight on the forearm placed along the floor.
- Slowly stretch the legs upwards to make the entire body perpendicular to the floor.
- Stay in this position for one to five minutes.
- Bend the knees and slowly come back to the knee-elbow position. Raise the head from the clasped hands and release the fingers.

Fig. 13: Shirshasana

Precautions

- This asana should be done slowly in stages and no jerky movements should be made.
- Obese individuals can do it by supporting their legs against the wall or by using a special apparatus easily available.
- People suffering from hypertension, heart diseases, eye diseases, ear diseases, cervical or lumbar spondylitis and kidney diseases should avoid this asana.
- It should not be practiced during pregnancy or menstruation.

(b) Mudras

Definition

Mudra is a psychic, emotional, devotional and aesthetic gesture or attitude. It is a combination of subtle physical movement which alters mood, attitude and perception and deepens awareness and concentration. It may involve the whole body as a part of an asana, pranayama, bandha or visualisation techniques or a simple posture of the hands.

Mudras lead to awakening of the pranas, chakras and kundalini and bestow major siddhis and psychic powers on the person who practices them.

Mudras Useful in Sleep Disorders

Gyana or Dhyana Mudra (Meditation)

Techniques

- Sit in a meditative posture like Padmasana or Sukhasana with eyes closed.
- Place the straightened hand on the knees with palms facing upwards. Touch the tip of thumb with the tip of index finger and keep the other fingers straight. Do this in both hands.
- Practice this mudra for at least 30 to 45 minutes twice a day starting with 5 to 10 minutes initially.

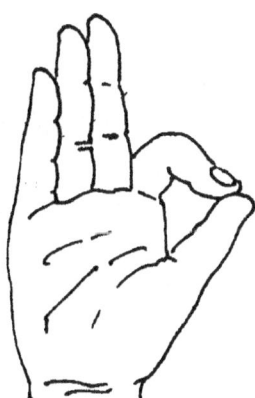

Fig. 14: Gyana Mudra

Prithvi Mudra (Earth Mudra)

Technique

- This consists of putting the tips of thumb and ring finger together. Keep other fingers straight. This mudra cures weakness of the body and makes the body robust, sturdy and full of vigour.

Kakimudra (Crow's Beak)

Technique

- ❑ Sit in any comfortable asana with the head and spine straight and hands resting on the knees in Gyana Mudra.
- ❑ Close the eyes and relax the whole body for a few minutes.
- ❑ Open the eyes and perform Nasikagra Drishti (mudra) by focussing both eyes on the tip of the nose.
- ❑ Purse the lips forming a beak through which air may be inhaled.
- ❑ Inhale slowly and deeply through pursed lips.
- ❑ Close the lips and exhale slowly through the nose.
- ❑ Repeat the procedure several times.

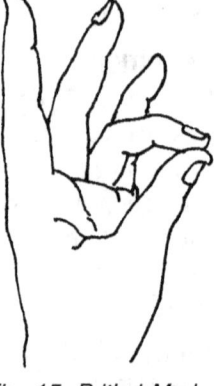

Fig. 15: Prithvi Mudra

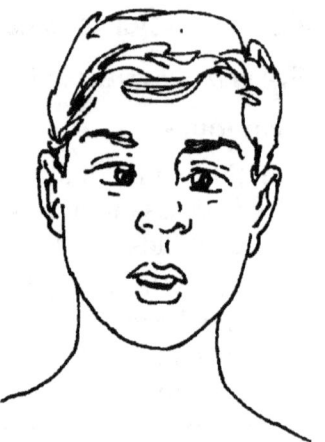

Fig. 16: Kakimudra

Precautions

- ❑ It should not be practiced in a polluted atmosphere or in excessively cold weather because the normal filtering and air conditioning function of the nose is bypassed.
- ❑ People suffering from depression, low blood pressure and chronic constipation should avoid this mudra.

Yoga Mudra

Technique

- Exhale slowly and bend the trunk forward keeping the hands at the back.
- Gradually bring the face down, the head touching the floor.
- Retain this posture as well as the breath for as long as possible.
- Relax the neck and back.
- Slowly exhale and come back to the original position.
- Repeat this three to five times.

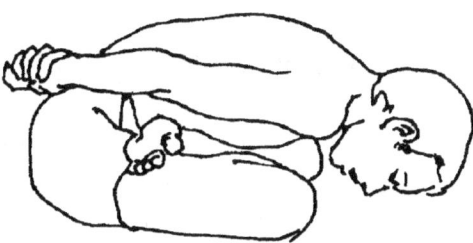

Fig 17: Yoga Mudra

Precautions

Those suffering from sciatica, hypertension, heart disease, pelvic inflammatory disease, hernia, duodenal ulcer following surgery should avoid this mudra.

Benefits of *mudras*

- Shunya Mudra can relieve earache in a few minutes.
- Apana Mudra can relieve urinary obstruction and other urinary problems within a few minutes.
- If Vayu Mudra and Apana Mudra are done together the acute pain in the chest and increased heart rate can be controlled within seconds.

- In trismus (difficulty in opening the mouth) when middle finger is rubbed with the thumb, there is a quick relief & the mouth opens.
- Similarly difficulty in closing the eyes or exophthalmos can be quickly controlled by Prana Mudra.
- Vayu Mudra can help in treating without medicines gout, hemiplegia (paralysis), tremors and other vague pains and neuropathies in the body.
- Stomachache can be quickly relieved by Apana Mudra.
- Bhujangini Mudra and Yoga Mudra improve the digestive system.
- Khechari Mudra stimulates the pituitary and pineal glands and improves memory.
- Ashwini Mudra prevents piles, prolapse of uterus and rectum. It controls gastritis and constipation.
- Yoga Mudra and Vajroli Mudra strengthens the prostate glands and reproductive organs.
- Maha Mudra keeps the heart muscle active and strengthens the functions of the prostate and seminal vesicles.
- Pashini Mudra stimulates the nervous system, reduces excess fat, controls diabetes and improves digestion.
- Hridaya Mudra is very beneficial for heart ailments, especially coronary heart disease.
- Shambhvi Mudra, Nasikagra Mudra and Bhoochari Mudra strengthen the eye muscles and remove emotional stress and anger, developing concentra-tion and mental stability.
- Shanmukhi Mudra is useful in the treatment of infections of the eyes, ears, nose and throat.
- Viparceta Karni Mudra improves blood circulation to the abdominal organs, brain, lungs and heart.

(c) Yogic Kriyas

Yogic Kriyas are a very important aspect of Hatha Yoga as they help to eliminate the accumulated toxins from the body. As in the case of a machine, the body has to be continuously cleaned and maintained. The Yogic Kriyas are six in number and often referred to as *Shat Kriyas* or *Shat Karma*. These are as follows:-

- Neti
- Kapalbhati
- Dhauti
- Nauli
- Basti
- Trataka

Kriyas useful for sleep disorders

Neti

Neti is a process that helps to clean the nasal passages. This is of three types:

- Sutraneti or Rubberneti
- Jalaneti
- Ghritha Neti or Ghee drops

Sutraneti or Rubberneti

Technique

- A cotton string stiffened with wax or a rubber catheter of numbers three, four or five is used.
- It is slowly inserted through one nostril with right hand and gradually pulled out through the mouth with the left hand.

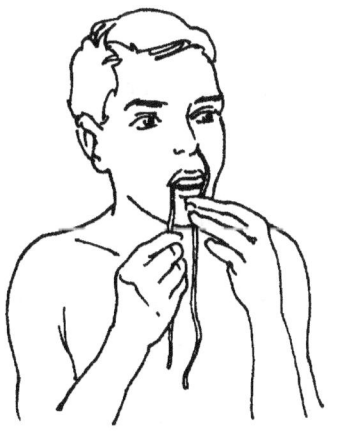

Fig 18: Sutraneti

- Then both the ends are moved forwards & backwards in the nostril about 15-20 times.
- Remove the string through the mouth and repeat the same procedure for the other nostril.
- This procedure is done once daily initially and after one month reduced to twice or thrice a week.

Precautions
- This procedure is to be strictly done under the guidance of an expert.
- Persons with high blood pressure, bleeding from nose, deviated nasal septum and severe cold should not practise this kriya.
- Finger nails should be properly cut and hands washed with soap and water.
- Spectacles if any should be removed before practising Neti.
- In the beginning of Neti, when the thread or catheter is introduced there may be an itching sensation in the nostrils with sneezing and watering from the eyes. These symptoms will subside with regular practice.

Jalaneti

This is another technique of nasal cleansing using salt water instead of thread or catheter.

Technique
- Boil about a litre of water in a vessel and allow it to cool.
- Add a teaspoonful of salt to it and stir well.
- Transfer this water to a Jalaneti pot.
- Stand erect, step forward and insert the spout gently into one of the nostrils.

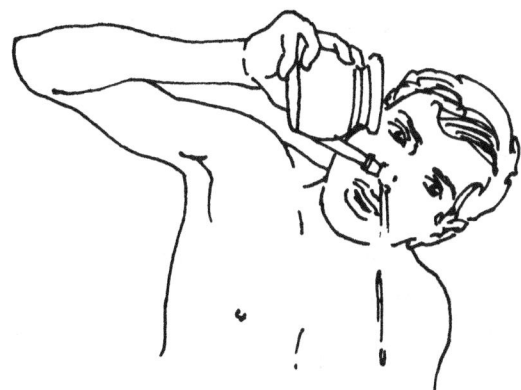

Fig 19: Jalaneti

- ❑ Slowly tilt the head to the other side so that water runs into one nostril and comes out of the other.
- ❑ Keep the mouth open and breathe normally through the mouth.
- ❑ Allow water to flow freely through the other nostril continuously like a stream.
- ❑ Repeat the procedure for the other nostril.
- ❑ This procedure should be done once daily or more often if one is suffering from cold and stuffy nose.

Precautions

- ❑ The concentration of salt and the temperature of water should be maintained evenly throughout the practice.
- ❑ The nozzle of Jalneti pot should not be inserted too deeply into the nostril since it may injure the sensitive lining of the nose.
- ❑ Do not inhale through the nose or else the salt water will enter the mouth.
- ❑ In the beginning of the procedure there may be itching or irritation in the nose, sneezing or watering of the eyes. This will improve with practice.
- ❑ The nose should be dried properly after the procedure since water left off may cause cold and sinusitis. This can be done by moving the head in different directions and exhaling forcibly.

- ❏ This procedure should not be done after meals.
- ❏ Do not blow the nose too hard since the water may be pushed into the ears.

Ghrithaneti

Technique

Pure desi ghee prepared from cow's milk is applied in the form of nasal drops. This ghee is to be warmed until it liquefies and then with the help of dropper one-two drops of it is applied into each nostril. After applying ghee, cover the face with a towel and rub the area around the nose. Ghrithaneti should be done before doing Sutraneti and Jalneti.

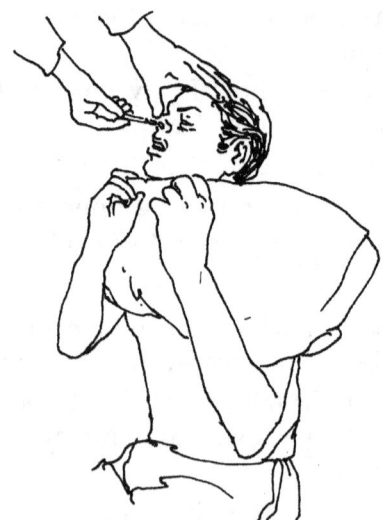

Fig. 20: Ghrithaneti

Kunjal Kriya or Vamana Dhauti

Technique

- ❏ Take about one litre of lukewarm water flavoured with aniseed and cardamom.

- Drink this water as quickly as possible till a vomiting sensation is felt.
- Stand up immediately, bend forward and insert first three fingers of the right hand into the mouth and tickle the uvula till vomiting is induced.
- Continue this process till all the water comes out.
- This can be repeated once a week.

Precautions

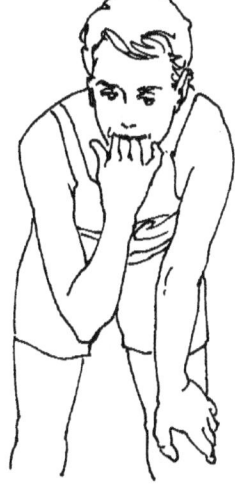

Fig. 21: Kunjal Kriya

- This procedure should be done only in the early morning on an empty stomach.
- Food should not be taken for at least half an hour after practice.
- Finger nails should be trimmed well and hands washed with soap and water before performing this procedure.
- People suffering from stomach ulcer, eye diseases, heart problems, stroke, hernia should avoid this kriya.

Trataka (concentrated gazing)

Trataka is an eye exercise which is done by focusing the eye on a selected object.

Technique

- Sit in a comfortable meditative posture with the head, neck and back erect and the body relaxed.

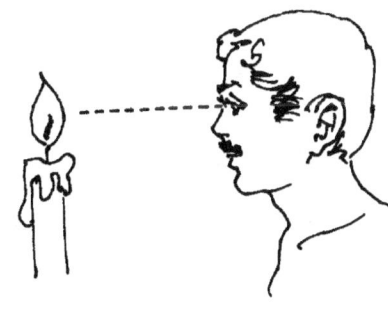

Fig. 22: Trataka

- Place a lighted candle on a table at the level of the eyes at a distance of about one to two feet from the face.
- Open the eyes and gaze intently at the brightest spot of the flame just above the wick.
- Continue gazing at the spot of the flame with total concentration without moving the eyeballs or blinking and without any awareness of the rest of the body.
- Initially gaze for two to three minutes, then close your eyes.
- Try to visualise the after-image of the candle flame in front of closed eyes.
- When this image of the candle disappears, open the eyes and again start gazing the flame tip.
- Increase the duration of gazing each time and do it for maximum possible period.

Precautions

- Trataka should preferably be done at dawn or dusk when the stomach is empty.
- For insomnia this should be practiced for 10 to 15 minutes before going to sleep.
- Trataka should be performed after asanas and pranayama
- It should be practiced on a steady flame with no draught of air in the vicinity.
- Undue strain to the eyes should be avoided.
- In case of eye diseases like myopia, astigmatism and early cataract, a black dot of about 0.5 cm in diametre should be used instead of a candle flame.
- Epileptics should practice trataka on a totally steady object.
- Avoid practicing trataka on the sun since the delicate membranes of eyes may be damaged. Also avoid

doing trataka on the moon, a crystal ball, a mirror or darkness.
- While gazing if the concentration is disturbed by suppressed thoughts or emotions, this practice should be stopped immediately.
- The object for gazing should not be changed since the mind will take time to adapt to the new object.

Kapalbhati (frontal brain cleansing)

Kapalbhati is basically a form of pranayama though older yogic texts have classified it as a part of Shatkarmas. It is of three types:

  i) Vatkarma Kapalbhati
  ii) Vyutkarma Kapalbhati
  iii) Sheetkarma Kapalbhati

i) Vatkarma Kapalbhati

Technique
- Sit in any comfortable asana with the head and spine straight and the hands resting on the knees.
- Close the eyes and relax the whole body.
- Inhale deeply through both nostrils expanding the abdomen and exhale with a forceful contraction of the abdominal muscles, making a hissing noise.
- The next inhalation takes place by passively allowing the abdominal muscles to expand spontaneously without any effort.
- After completing 10 rapid breaths in succession, inhale and exhale deeply completing one round.
- Complete three to five such rounds.

Precautions
- The rapid breathing in this technique should be from the abdomen and not from the chest.

- It should be practiced after asanas or neti and preferably on an empty stomach or three to four hours after meals.
- If pain or giddiness is experienced, it should be stopped and cause found out.
- Kapalbhati should not be practiced by those suffering from heart disease, high blood pressure, vertigo, epilepsy, stroke, hernia or peptic ulcer.

ii) Vyutkarma Kapalbhati

Technique

- Fill a bowl with one litre of warm water, add two teaspoonfuls of salt and dissolve it well.
- Sit in a comfortable asane with head and spine straight.
- Scoop the water up in the palm of the hand and sniff it in through the nostrils.
- Let the water flow down to the mouth and then spit it out.
- Practice it several times.
- Dry the nostrils properly.

iii) Sheetkarma Kapalbhati

Technique

- Maintain the posture as in the Vyutkarma Kapalbhati.
- Take a mouthful of warm saline water.
- Suck it noisily through the mouth and expel it through nostrils.
- Repeat it several times.
- Dry the nostrils properly.

Precautions

- Vyutkarma and Sheetkarma Kapalbhati may be performed at any time of the day except immediately after meals.

- Before attempting these two techniques, jalneti should be done.
- People with nasal bleeding should not perform these two practices.
- If not done properly water may enter the lungs causing pneumonia.

How *yogic kriyas* help in sleep disorders?
- They help in eleminating of toxins like mucus, gas, acid, sweat, urine and stool.
- They improve the functioning of the excretory organs.
- They help keep the eyes, nose, sinuses, food pipe, and digestive system clean and tone up their functioning.
- These Kriyas help to build up resistance to diseases and sharpen the mind.
- They also help to prepare the body and condition it for proper practice of Yogasanas, Pranayama, Yoga nidra and meditation.
- These techniques are very useful in healing many psychosomatic disorders.

(d) Pranayama

Definition
Pranayama is derived from two sanskrit words – "Prana" and "Ayama". "Prana" means breath, life, vitality, air, power or energy. "Ayama" denotes extension, abstinence, regulation, control or restraint. Thus Pranayama is the act of control of respiration and an attempt to controlling the flow of "Prana" or vital force in the human body.

Stages of *Pranayama*
Pranayama consists of four stages:
1. The "Puraka" or Inhalation Phase: Slow sustained flow of inhalation.
2. The "Kumbhaka" or Breath-holding Phase: Controlled suspension and retention of breath after inhalation.

3. The "Rechaka" or Exhalation Phase: Slow and long controlled exhalation.
4. The "Shunyaka" or End of Breathing: Breath-holding after exhalation.

Rules for *Pranayama*
1. Pranayama is to be preferably practised in the open air or in a quiet, clean, well-ventilated room.
2. The best and most comfortable posture for Pranayama is Padmasana.
3. The place for such a practice is to be neat and clean and without any distraction.
4. Pranayama should not be practiced in a crowded place. It may be done on a river bank.
5. The best time for Pranayama is early morning when the air is pure and oxygen is available in abundance. If not possible, then it may be done in the evening after sunset.
6. Tight dress should not be used, but loose comfortable clothes.
7. One should not smoke atleast one hour before or after practice.
8. Pranayama should be done under the guidance of an expert, if possible.
9. It should be done after a good rest at night.
10. Breathing should be done through the nostrils only.
11. The breath-holding practice should not be done by heavy weight-lifters.
12. Pranayama should not be practiced while walking or lying.
13. There should be a gap of at least 3 hours between taking of medicine and beginning of Pranayama.
14. If one feels dizzy while practicing Pranayama, it should be stopped immediately.

15. Pranayama should be practiced after asanas and before meditation.
16. A bath may be taken before commencing the practice or at least the hands, face and feet must be washed. After Pranayama, the bath should not be taken for atleast half an hour to allow the body temperature to become normalize.
17. Pranayama should be done on an empty stomach or three to four hours after a meal.
18. No undue strain should be applied as lungs are very delicate organs and can be easily injured.
19. Some individuals may exhibit certain symptoms while practicing pranayama, *i.e.* itching, tingling, heat or cold, feeling of heaviness, constipation or reduced urination. These symptoms usually disappear with regular practice. If symptoms persistent, a yoga expert may be consulted.

Benefits of *Pranayama*
1. Pranayama improves the functioning of the lungs through increased oxygenation of blood vessels of the lungs as well as all parts of the lungs.
2. It increases the capacity of the lungs to inhale and exhale air.
3. Breath-holding can train the body to function properly even in low oxygen levels.
4. The blood supply to the heart and brain is improved by Pranayama.
5. It enhances the concentration of mind and improves the relaxation of the body.
6. Pranayama cleans up and purifies the nose, nasal sinuses and respiratory passages.
7. The digestion is improved due to improved blood supply and pressure of the diaphragm in the abdominal organs.

8. Plavini Pranayama is believed to exert control over hunger and thirst in the individual who practices it.

Useful *Pranayamas* for sleep disorders

i) Nadi Shodhana Pranayama or Anuloma - Viloma

Technique

- ❑ Sit in any comfortable meditative posture preferably Padmasana keeping the head and spine upright.
- ❑ Close the eyes, relax the body and breathe freely for sometime.
- ❑ Rest the index and middle fingers gently in the centre of eyebrows and the thumb and ring finger above the right and left nostrils respectively. These two fingers control the flow of breath in the nostrils by alternately closing one nostril to block the flow of breath and while keeping the other nostril open. This is the Nasikagra Mudra.

Step - I

- ❑ Close the right nostril with the thumb and breathe in through the left nostril, counting silently 1,2,3. Similarly close the left nostril with the ring finger releasing pressure of thumb on the right nostril and breathe out, counting 1,2,3. The time for inhalation and exhalation should be equal.

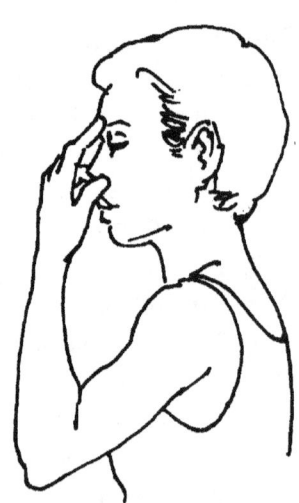

Fig. 23: Nadi Shodhana Pranayama

- ❑ Repeat the procedure by inhaling through the right nostril and exhaling through the left one. This makes up one round. Ten rounds are to be practiced.
- ❑ Slowly increase the counting up to 12:12 for inhalation/exhalation. This is followed by changing the ratio to

1:2, i.e. breathe in for count 5 and breathe out for count 10 adding up to ratio 12:24.

Step - II

After mastering Step-I, this step-II should be practiced.

- ❑ Close the right nostril and inhale through the left nostril for a count of 5. After this close both nostrils and retain air in the lungs for a count of 5. Then, open the right nostril, breathe in slightly and slowly breathe out for a count of 5.
- ❑ This is repeated by inhaling from the right nostril, retaining and breathing out from the left side. Repeat 10 times.
- ❑ Increase the ratio from 1:1:1 for inhalation, retention and exhalation to 1:2:2, 1:3:2 and 1:4:2.

Step-III

- ❑ In this step, inhalation is started from the left nostril as above, followed by retention (breath-holding) and exhalation from right nostril which is also followed by breath-holding.
- ❑ The procedure is also repeated as above by inhalation from the right nostril and 10 rounds to be done.
- ❑ The ratio is started as above 1:1:1:1 and increased to 1:4:2:2 and duration is also increased from a count of five to the maximum limit where comfortable.

Precautions

- ❑ Breathing should be free flowing and never forced.
- ❑ Breathing should never be done through the mouth.
- ❑ This technique of Pranayama is best done under the guidance of an expert.
- ❑ If there is any sign of discomfort, the procedure should be discontinued.
- ❑ The best time to practice is early morning after having performed the asanas.

- The duration of this Pranayama should be about 10 to 15 minutes daily comprising 5 to 10 rounds.
- Patients suffering from hypertension and heart disease must avoid breath-holding in this Pranayama.

ii) Sheetali Pranayama

Technique

- Sit in any comfortable meditative posture with hands on the knees as in Gyana Mudra.
- Close the eyes and relax the whole body.
- Draw the tongue outside the mouth and roll it up from the sides to form a channel like a bird's beak.
- Slowly and deeply inhale the air through it and fill the lungs completely.
- After complete inhalation, withdraw the tongue, close the mouth and exhale through the nose.
- Repeat the exercise 5 to 10 times.
- Gradually increase the rounds up to 15 or even more as well as the duration of each inhalation/exhalation.

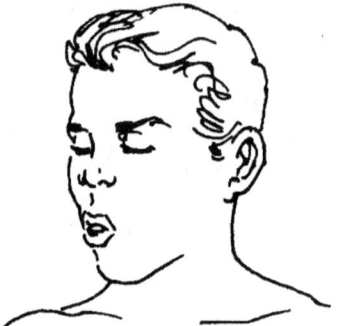

Fig. 24: Sheetali Pranayama

Precautions

- This technique should not be practiced in a dirty, polluted atmosphere since breathing such air through the mouth transfers it directly into the lungs.
- This Pranayama is not suitable for patients suffering from low blood pressure or respiratory disorders, such as asthma and bronchitis.
- People with constipation should also avoid this Pranayama.

- ❑ Sheetali Pranayama should be avoided in winter or in cold climates.
- ❑ It should be practiced after asanas and other yogic practices which produce heat in the body; in order to restore the balance of temperature.

iii) Sheetkari Pranayama

Technique

- ❑ Sit in any comfortable position with the hands on the knees.
- ❑ Close the eyes and relax the whole body.
- ❑ Hold the teeth lightly together, keeping the lips open.
- ❑ Slightly press the tip of the tongue against the lower front teeth and then inhale the air slowly through the mouth over the tongue with a hissing sound.
- ❑ After full inhalation withdraw the tongue and close the mouth and slowly exhale through both nostrils.
- ❑ Complete 5 to 10 rounds.

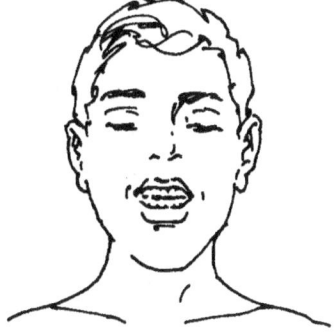

Fig. 25: Sheetkari Pranayama

Precaution

- ❑ As with Sheetali Pranayama, people with infected teeth and gums, missing teeth or denture should not practise this Pranayama.

Benefits

As for Sheetali Pranayama, along with the additional advantage, it keeps the teeth and gums healthy.

iv) Bhramari Pranayama

Technique

- Sit in a comfortable meditative posture with eyes closed, head and spine erect and hand resting on the knees.
- Close the eyes and relax the whole body completely for a short time.

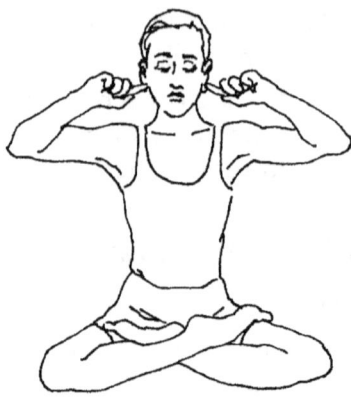

Fig 26: Bhramari Pranayama

- The lips should remain gently closed with the teeth slightly separated and jaws completely relaxed.
- Raise the arms sideways and bend the elbows, bringing the hands to the ears and plugging each ear with the index or middle finger.
- Inhale thoroughly with lungs full, through the nostrils.
- Exhale slowly and in a controlled manner while making a deep, steady humming sound like that of black bee.
- Repeat the procedure 5 to 10 times.

Precautions

- It can be practiced at any time provided the surrounding is quiet and peaceful.
- It should not be performed while lying down.
- People suffering from severe ear infections should not practice this Pranayama.

v) Ujjayi Pranayama

Technique

- Sit in any comfortable meditative posture.
- Close the eyes and relax the whole body.

- Inhale slowly and deeply through both the nostrils with a low, uniform frictional sound through the glottis and expand the chest naturally.
- Hold the breath for sometime.
- Then exhale through both the nostrils.
- Relax the chest for a few seconds before going into the next round.
- Practice for 10 to 20 minutes.

Precautions
- Care should be taken to see that the abdomen does not expand during inhalation.
- Breath-holding should not be done by patients of heart disease.
- Do not contract the throat or facial muscles strongly.
- People with spondylitis or a slipped disc can practice it in Vajrasana or Makarasana.

vi) Bhastrika Pranayama

Technique
- Sit in any comfortable meditative posture with hands resting on the knees in Gyana Mudra.
- Keep the head and spine straight, close the eyes and relax the whole body.
- Using Nasikagra Mudra close the right nostril with the thumb.
- Breathe in and out forcefully through the left nostril for about 10 times. The abdomen should expand and contract rhythmically with the breath.
- Now close the left nostril and breathe rapidly and forcefully through the right nostril.
- Similarly breathing can be done through both the nostrils simultaneously.
- At the end of each procedure, breath-holding may be done for up to 30 seconds.

Precautions

- During Bhastrika, only the abdomen should move and not the chest or shoulders.
- The breathing sound should only appear from the abdomen and not the throat or chest.
- If there is a feeling of giddiness, vomiting or excessive perspiration, Bhastrika should be stopped.
- Violent respiration, facial contortions and excessive shaking of the body should be avoided.
- Bhastrika should not be practiced by people suffering from hypertension, heart disease, duodenal ulcer, hernia, stroke, epilepsy or vertigo.
- Neti may be practiced if there is blockage of nostrils with mucus.

vii) Moorchha Pranayama

Technique

- Sit in any comfortable meditative asanas with the head and spine straight and the whole body relaxed.
- Breathe slowly and deeply for sometime.
- Fold the tongue upward and backward so that the lower surface lies in contact with the palate (Khechari Mudra).
- Then slowly inhale through both nostrils as in Ujjayi Pranayama.
- Gently bend the head slightly back and look upward and inward focusing the eyes at the centre of eyebrows. Hold the gaze for a few seconds (Shambhavi Mudra).

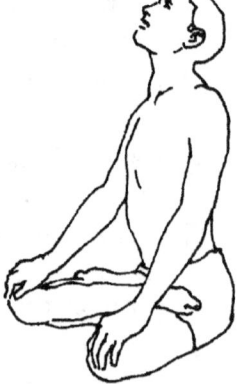

Fig. 27: Moorchha Pranayam

- Keeping the arms straight by locking the elbows and pressing the knees with the hands, retain the breath for as long as possible maintaining Shambhavi Mudra.
- Exhale, relax the arms, close the eyes and bring back the head to the upright position.
- Relax the whole body with the eyes closed.

Precautions
- This Pranayama should be done under the guidance of an expert.
- Persons with high blood pressure, heart disease, epilepsy and brain disorders should avoid it.
- Do not continue if fainting sensation is felt.

(e) What is Yoga Nidra?

Yoga Nidra is a form of Raja Yoga in which awareness is progressively withdrawn from everything: the external surroundings, ¾ the body, the breathing, the conscious and the unconscious mind. It is a state of mind between wakefulness and sleep. It opens the deeper phase of the mind, inducing complete physical, mental and emotional relaxation.

Yoga Nidra is a more efficient and effective form of psychic and physiological rest and more rejuvenating than conventional sleep. A single hour of Yoga Nidra is equivalent to four hours of conventional sleep.

Prerequisites for doing Yoga Nidra

1. It should be done in a quiet room with doors and windows closed.
2. The television, radio, music system etc should be off.
3. The room should be well ventilated, neither hot nor cold, with no cold draft of air (A.C./cooler) directed towards the body.
4. The room should preferably be dark with curtains drawn.

5. The person should wear light, loose clothing.
6. The person should lie in Shavasana with eyes closed, palms facing upwards, arms away from the body and legs about 30 to 35 cm apart and head, neck and spine straight.
7. Yoga Nidra should be initially done under the guidance of an experienced teacher and later independently.
8. It should be done on an empty stomach or about 3 hours after a meal or half an hour after light refreshments.
9. The person should not fall asleep while doing Yoga Nidra.
10. Initially it should be done for 5 to 10 minutes and in a few days increased up to 45 minutes.
11. Pain or stiffness in the body can be relieved by doing Yogasanas before performing Yoga Nidra.

Procedure

Yoga Nidra is practiced in different stages as given below.

Stage I–Preparation for Yoga Nidra

This involves following instructions as given above.

Stage II–Relaxation of the body

Initially listen to the sounds in the distance and become aware of each sound without trying to find out the source. Then move the attention to sounds in the room. Visualize the body from the head to toes and be aware of the normal breathing. Silently repeat the mantra "Om" and also "I am aware, I am going to practice Yoga Nidra."

Stage III–Resolution or Sankalpa

In this stage, a resolve or resolution should be made. It should be a short, positive statement in simple language, stated thrice with awareness, feeling and emphasis.

The resolution or "Sankalpa" made during Yoga Nidra will surely become true in life. The resolution can be materialistic, mental or spiritual. It may be one of these:

"I will be successful in my efforts."

"I will be more efficient."

"I will achieve normal health."

"I will help others positively."

"I will awaken my spiritual potential."

Stage IV—Rotation of consciousness on body parts

Without moving any part of the body initially visualise and become aware of each part of the body in a systematic manner. Start from right thumb and say mentally "right thumb", then move to index finger, middle finger, ring finger, little finger, palm, back of the hand, wrist, forearm, elbow, arm, shoulder, armpit, waist, hip, thigh, knee, leg, ankle, foot, sole, right big toe, second toe, third toe, fourth toe, little toe. Repeat the same on the left side followed by other parts of the body on the back and the front of the body. Do not open the eyes or shift the gaze to the specific part of the body.

Stage V—Awareness of breathing

Be aware of the breathing through the nostrils. Concentrate on the breathing through each nostril. Concentrate on the movements of the chest and abdomen during inspiration and expiration. Silently count the respiration from 50 to zero or any other numbers.

Stage VI—Awareness of sensations and emotions

Feel the different sensations in different parts of the body, *e.g.* heat and cold, heaviness and lightness, pain and pleasure, joy and sorrow, love and hate etc.

Stage VII—Visualisation of images

Visualise an image as described in detail by the instructor. It may be a landscape, an ocean, a mountain, temple, flower, riverbank, a rising sun, a saint, chakras, lingam, cross or a golden egg.

This brings out the hidden content of the unconscious mind to the conscious level. It develops self-awareness and will power and relaxes the mind by purging out disturbing thoughts.

Stage VIII–Completion
Become aware of the breathing and the whole body lying on the floor from the head to toes. Repeat "Om" silently twice more. Visualise the floor, the position of the body, the room and its surroundings. Repeat the resolution and have faith that it will become true. Slowly open your eyes and move the body and stretch yourself and sit down. This completes the practice of Yoga Nidra.

Benefits of Yoga Nidra
1. Yoga Nidra is a successful treatment for insomnia producing definite decrease in the time required to fall asleep. Those who practise it at bedtime report that they fall asleep even before completing the practice. It can induce sleep without dependence on any sedative or hypnotic.
2. Other diseases where Yoga Nidra is useful are hypertension, heart diseases, asthma, peptic ulcer, arthritis, migraine, anxiety, depression and drug addiction.

(f) Meditation
Definition
Patanjali, the original teacher of yoga, had described meditation as "the uninterrupted thinking of one thought." Swami Vivekananda had said, "Meditation is the focus of the mind on some object. If the mind acquires concentration on one object it can concentrate on any object whatsoever."

Basic procedure of meditation
Though different religions, communities and sects may have some variation on the procedure of meditation, the

basic procedure is almost similar in all cases. The main goal in meditation is to withdraw the mind and senses from the surrounding environment and focus the attention on any given object.

Meditation is usually done in the following steps.

Complete relaxation

Complete relaxation refers to the conscious suspension of all movements of the body resulting in relaxation of all skeletal muscles and limpness of the body. Adopting either sitting postures like Padmasana, Sukhasana and Vajrasana or the standing posture:

- maintain the posture and keep the spine and neck straight and the whole body relaxed.
- concentrate your mind on each part of the body one by one starting from the toe to the head.
- allow each part to relax and feel that it has become relaxed completely.

Awareness of breathing

- Concentrate completely on the breathing, taking slow, deep and rhythmic breaths.
- Concentrate at the meeting point of both nasal cavities and perceive both the incoming and outgoing breaths.
- Next concentrate on the navel and be fully aware of the contraction and expansion of abdominal muscles during exhalation and inhalation respectively.
- Alternate breathing can also be practiced during meditation without causing any wandering thoughts or discomfort.

Awareness of body parts

- Concentrate on each part of the body one by one perceiving the sensations and vibrations in each part. Start with the big toe of right foot, moving upwards in the front and back to the head focussing on each part.

❏ Perceive the body as a whole while assuming or even standing up slowly from the sitting posture.

Awareness of chakras or psychic centres

❏ While sitting in the relaxed posture, focus the attention on the seven chakras or psychic centres, starting from the Muladhara Chakra or Shakti Kendra.

❏ Imagine as if the vibrations are flowing from Muladhara Chakra upwards up to Sahasra Chakra or Jyoti Kendra.

Awareness of psychic colours

The chakras or psychic centres can be activated by visualising certain colours which are capable of producing specific vibrations. This is possible by regular practice of meditation.

❏ While perceiving the different chakras or psychic centres, one should visualise a particular colour which is specific for it. This helps in activating these centres and enhancing their physiological functions.

Auto-suggestion and resolution

Auto-suggestion refers to the repeated recitation of a sentence, *e.g.* "The pain in my knee is disappearing" or "My headache has gone" etc. Auto-suggestion helps in building up the faith and belief and the tolerance to bear the disease or its effects. This also brings up physiological changes in the body by weakening the forces of disease, mental imbalance and emotional disturbances.

Resolution or contemplation refers to building up healthy and positive attitude towards life. This can be done by repeating "I will not steal" or "I will tell the truth"' or "I will stand first in the class" etc. Repetition of such a resolution helps in overcoming negative attitudes and psychological distortions and develops positive attitudes like truthfulness, amity, fearlessness, tolerance, love, sympathy etc.

Benefits of meditation in sleep disorders
1. It brings about calmness in the mind, controlling disturbing thoughts.
2. It controls negative emotions and brings about a positive thinking.
3. It acts as a natural tranquilliser bringing about a deep and natural sleep.
4. Nightmares, night terrors and excessive dreaming are overcome.
5. Mental disorders like anxiety, depression, schizophrenia can be treated with regular practice of meditation.
6. Blood pressure is brought under control in people with hypertension.
7. Stabilises the neuromuscular, neuroendocrine and immunological systems, help in keeping the body and mind healthy and harmonious and stress is weeded out.
8. Regular practice of meditation leads to introspection of self and perception of reality of life and its associated problems. This helps people avoid situations or circumstances which disturb the biological rhythm or emotional harmony which leads to tranquility and peace of mind.

5. Naturopathy

Role of Naturopathy in Treatment
Naturopathy or Nature Cure is the technique of following the rules of nature and exploring the natural resources, like the sun, air, water and soil, to cure various maladies.

The branches of Naturopathy useful for the treatment of sleep disorders are as follows:

1. Hydrotherapy
2. Mud Therapy
3. Massage

1. Hydrotherapy

Water is very essential for our life. It not only quenches our thirst but also has certain medicinal properties by virtue of its rich mineral content. Water contains copper, carbon, sulphur, phosphorus, iodine, calcium and other valuable minerals and chemicals of medicinal value. There are many appliances which are more attractive and effective. These are sauna bath, jet bath, circular jet bath, hip bath, foot bath, arm bath, turkish bath, douches, water vibration, irrigation, whirlpool bath.

How does hydrotherapy work in sleep disorders?

- Hot water is useful in relieving internal and deep congestion. It increases the blood circulation and body heat.
- Cold water is useful in reducing swelling and superficial congestion. It relaxes blood vessels and normalises blood circulation and body temperature.
- Water reduces inflammation.
- Water relieves pain.
- It increases blood circulation of sluggish organs of body.
- It eliminates toxins from the body.
- It lowers or raises the temperature of the body.

Types of hydrotherapy useful for sleep disorders

Cold spinal bath: A specially designed tub called spinal bath tub is used for this bath. The side of the tub is slightly elevated so that the patient can keep his head on it comfortably. This tub is made up of zinc. Three types of water temperatures are used in this bath. They are (1) Cold Spinal bath (2) Neutral and (3) Hot Spinal bath.

Method: The temperature of the bath is maintained at 55ºF to 65ºF by pouring cold water in the tub. The depth of the water is 2 to 2 ½". The patient is asked to lie down inside the tub with the head on the elevated side and the legs on the small stool. Both hands can be kept on either side of the tub by the sides of the body in the water. The duration of the bath can be from 10-20 minutes depending on the necessity.

In the absence of a spinal tub, a cold wet compress or a long rubber bag filled with cold water or ice can be applied to the entire spine. It will serve the same effect as that of cold spinal bath. After the Spinal bath the water should be wiped out immediately and the patient asked to bathe for 10-15 minutes. In case of weak patients, he is advised to lie on the bed covered with a blanket and bath to be taken after 30 minutes.

Physiological effects

Cold water is useful in reducing swelling & superficial congestion. It relaxes blood vessels & normalises blood circulation and body temperature.

Therapeutic effects

It is useful in relieving the congestion of brain, various types of vomiting, epilepsy, hysteria, insomnia, fever, constipation, sunstroke etc. Cold Spinal bath is also useful in extreme irritability of the body *e.g.* burning sensation on the back in chronic eczema & psoriasis where there is no discharge.

Contra-indications

In sciatica, paralysis, asthma, bronchitis, spondylitis, common cold, cough, backache & colics, such as uterine & renal colic, it is not applicable.

Neutral Spinal bath

Method/Procedure: It is same as that of cold bath. The temperature of water is maintained between 92°F to 98°F. Duration can vary between 15-60 minutes.

Therapeutic effects

It releases the nerve centres in the spinal bath, thus giving a calm & soothing effect on the viscera through the nerve filaments. It relieves nervous irritability & congestion of the brain & nervous system & cardiovascular system. It is very useful in cases of hypertension, insomnia & epilepsy.

Spray Spinal bath

This is an important bath for the treatment of diseases of the brain and spinal cord.

A spinal tub has been designed by Dr. Laxmana Sharma of Pudukottai, Tamil Nadu. This consists of a fibreglass tub with a perforated tube at the centre of the tub and a tank inside the tub having capacity of 40 litres. This tank is connected with a pipe to a 0.5 H.P. motor adjusted below the tub.

Ask the patient to lie down in the tub and start the machine. There will be a constant spray of ascending jet which will give a gentle massage to the whole spinal cord.

This is the most comfortable tub and also helps regulate temperature of water, *i.e.* cold, warm or neutral.

Therapeutic value of spinal spray

1. This procedure controls all the organs of the body, since most of the nerve roots start from the spinal cord. They are the sensory centres, temperature controlling centres, vasomotor centre and sympathetic & parasympathetic centres in the brain and spinal cord.
2. The neutral spinal spray is useful for insomnia, poor memory, fits, hysteria, mental retardation, tension, alcoholism etc. The cold spinal spray is beneficial in anxiety, irritability, hypertension, mania and excitement.

3. The small and large blood vessels of the heart, lungs, digestive system and brain contract (warm) or dilate (cold) depending on the temperature of water used in the spray. It improves oxygen supply to the lungs and heart by increasing blood circulation.
4. The warm or neutral spinal bath soothes the nerves and is an ideal form of hydrotherapy for insomnia. It relieves the tension of the muscles and nerves after exercise or after a day's hard work.
5. The warm spray can also stimulate the nerves relieving the pain of cervical spondylitis, low back pain, sciatica, and gastric and intestinal disturbances.

Precautions

Very hot spinal spray can give rise to burn in the skin.

Hot Foot bath

This is the most useful and effective form of water treatment for many disorders.

Procedures

A tub is filled with hot water in the temperature ranging from 102°F to 122°F depending on the tolerance of the individual. Alternately the temperature may be gradually increased after every 2-3 minutes. The duration of the bath ranges from10-20 minutes. Before starting the bath the individual is asked to drink 1 to 2 glasses of water. A wet towel is kept on the head. After the bath the feet must be kept in cold water for 1-2 minutes or rubbed with cold water using a towel followed by brisk drying with a thick towel.

Physiological effects

Hot foot bath dilates the blood vessels of the skin in the feet and draws blood from the congested parts of the body. By its reflex action it removes congestion from organs like the brain, lungs and genital organs.

Therapeutic effects

It is useful in headaches of all types, insomnia, fatigue, mental tiredness, poor blood circulation, rheumatism, sinusitis, asthma, bronchitis, menstrual problems, renal colic, gout, neuralgia etc.

Contraindications
It is not applicable in high fever, hypertension, cardiac ailments, pregnancy, menstrual period, prolonged fasting, fracture in legs etc.

2. Mud Therapy
The medicinal use of mud or clay is found in various conditions, especially in skin diseases. A poultice made of clay is a freely available natural treatment for many diseases and painful conditions. About 80% of surgical cases can be successfully treated by mud therapy.

Uses of mud therapy in sleep disorder
Mud therapy is useful for the following conditions which upon improvement induces good sleep:

1. Constipation—In case of simple constipation, apply warm mud pack on the abdomen in the evening before dinner or two to three hours after lunch or at night for ½ an hour or throughout the night.
2. Piles—Constipation is to be treated by the above method followed by the mud pack on the buttocks. In case of swelling, pain and bleeding, mud pack is to be cooled properly with ice and applied. This may be applied 10-12 times in case of severe pain or otherwise throughout night.
3. Dysentery—A thick cotton cloth soaked in lukewarm water and water squeezed out of it is applied to the abdomen. This is followed by fomentation with hot water bottle for 20-25 minutes. To this apply a warm mud pack for 30 minutes. After removing the mud pack, apply mustard oil on the abdomen and apply a warm cloth. Repeat this procedure three-four times. A butter-milk enema may be given after one-two mud packs.

4. Nocturnal emissions—Apply mud pack on the lower abdomen and penis along with enema until the problem is controlled.
5. Impotence—To the penis apply mud pack at night before going to sleep.
6. Insomnia—Warm mud pack should be applied on the neck and lower abdomen and enema should be taken. The sleeping environment should be clean and silent. While lying down chant Gayatri Mantra and concentrate on the breathing. Also feel the movements of the chest and abdomen while breathing. This will definitely put you to sleep.
7. Insanity—A cold mud pack on the head and hot pack on the abdomen for two-three times daily gives good results in a few days.
8. Simple fever—A cold mud pack is applied after every ½ hour on the abdomen about four-eight times depending on the need. Enema using lukewarm water can be given.
9. High grade fever—A cold mud pack is applied on the abdomen, head & forehead after every five minutes. If there is rigor with chills then avoid mud pack. Instead give hot water for drinking as well as for enema.
10. Headache—Apply wet clay on the head two-three times daily. In case of chronic headache, apply warm mud pack on the lower abdomen and back of the neck along with enema. Light diet should be taken along with this treatment.
11. Migraine—Wet mud pack to be applied on the head neck and throat.
12. For eye diseases—Apply wet clay pack on the eyes. Taking care to see that mud does not enter the eyes. Apply warm mud pack on the lower abdomen and behind the neck. This is a useful treatment for infections and inflammation of the eyes and even early cataract.
13. Skin diseases affecting face—pimples, white spots etc. —Mud pack with Multani Mitti is to be applied

on the face. After the mud dries, it should be washed with warm water, never with soap.

14. Mouth ulcers—Gopi chandan, a type of white clay, is to be applied after rubbing it on a flat surface with little water. Constipation is to be treated.
15. Mumps—Black clay from the fields or black silt is used for applying in the neck. This is very useful for treatment of mumps.
16. Diseases of the ears—Fill the ear partly with cotton followed by wet clay. Apply warm mud pack outside the affected ear as well as around the neck and throat. This is useful for the treatment of pain in the ear, boil inside the ear, discharge from the ear etc. In acute cases, mud therapy should be preceded by fomentation of ear with cloth soaked in hot water. Mud pack is to be changed repeatedly.
17. Diseases of the throat—A warm mud pack around the throat and neck is very useful for diseases of the throat.

How to use the mud?

1. Spread the mud in the hot sunlight and allow it to dry. If it is very sticky in nature add some sand to make it fine. Sieve it well and remove stones, dirt etc. In case of mud containing a lot of stones, dissolve in water, filter with a clean cloth and dry the filtrate. For good results, dissolve mud with water in a mud container overnight or one-two hours before usage.
2. Always use mud with a clean stick or spatula & never with hands.
3. In summer, mud should be dissolved in ice or cold water for better results.
4. For warm mud pack, boil water well and to it add mud.
5. Mud which is dissolved in water overnight should be well covered to avoid contamination by dirt, dust, stones etc.

6. Never re-use the mud which has been used for mud therapy.

Types of mud pack

1. Lower abdomen pack—This involves the application of mud pack from the level of umbilicus (navel) to the penis. Average size of mud pack is one inch long, eight inch broad and half an inch, thick but in obese individuals, the length and breadth is larger while in children it is smaller.

   Sometimes, the pack may be extended to the back also using a thick cloth which surrounds the lower abdomen and back.

2. Full abdomen pack—This may involve either the whole abdomen from below the ribs to the penis in front or both in the front and back.

3. Spine pack—This should be as long as the spine and more than 1" longer than the spine on both sides.

4. Chest pack—This starts from the throat to the lower end of ribs. Sometimes it may be extended in a circular fashion to the back also.

5. Throat pack—The size depends on the dimensions of the throat.

6. Ears pack—This involves applying mud pack from the chin to ½" above the ear.

7. Eyes pack—This should be from the nose to the forehead from one ear to the other about ½" thick.

8. Forehead pack—From above the eyes to the forehead and extending to both ears.

9. Head pack—Covering the whole head ½" thick like a cap.

10. Whole body pack—Use a thick bedsheet and apply wet mud on it. Then cover the whole body with the blanket in such a way that the mud spreads all over the body. Another bedsheet or blanket can be applied above the first bedsheet. Another way is to dig a pit

upto the size of the patient. Cover with wet mud and make patient lie with head & neck uncovered.

11. Lower abdominal pack—Extending from below the penis to lower abdomen & sidewards.
12. Penis pack—As above but involving penis two inches above and 2" thick.
13. For boil—Whole area surrounding boil for two inches long & ½" thick.

How to use mud therapy?

1. Apply mud pack for 30-60 minutes.
2. When the mud pack becomes warm its thickness should be increased. If it does not become warm in 1 hour, decrease the thickness.
3. Apply mud pack directly on the naked body and not above the clothes.
4. After applying a mud pack cover the body with an old cotton or wool cloth depending on the weather conditions.
5. After removing the pack, clean the area with a wet cloth and rub well with a dry towel for warming up the area.
6. For best results apply hot fomentation to the affected area before applying mud pack. This should not be done when high fever is present. Also a five minute and two minute cold & warm fomentation alternately is also useful for applying mud therapy.
7. Mud therapy is ideal for half an hour before enema & a walk.
8. The time of mud therapy is two hours before and three-four hours after a meal for abdomen pack. Other places except for chest, one hour after meals is also ideal.
9. It is very good to apply a mud pack before going to sleep.
10. For boils and injury regular mud pack changes hourly for one-two days is essential.

11. For wet wounds, eczema etc. a cold wet bandage pack is to be used and washed regularly with water boiled with neem leaves.

3. Massage

Massage is an excellent form of passive exercise. It tones up the nervous system. Improves breathing and quickens the elimination of toxins and waste material from the body. This is done through the various organs of elimination or excretion such as lungs, kidney, bowel and skin. It also boosts up the blood circulation and metabolic activities.

The massage techniques useful for sleep disorders are:

  i) Stroking
 ii) Circular kneading
iii) Pressure vibration

i) Stroking

For the treatment of insomnia and other sleep disorders slow and deep stroking of the spine is recommended. It involves using finger tips of both hands slowly but with some pressure and continuously from the neck (occiput) to the lower end of spine (sacrum). This movement not only relaxes the tightened and painful muscles but also the spinal nerves which in turn produce a sedative effect in the brain.

The massage should be given only on the sides of the vertebral column and not on the bones of the spines.

ii) Circular kneading

Using one or both hands rhythmically and slowly down the length of the spine, the soft tissues are pressed in a circular direction. For this the palm of the hand and fingers are used and not the back of the hand. No pressure should be applied on the bony spines.

This technique improves the circulation to the muscles and nerves of vertebral column and improves their nutrition and function. The muscles and nerves of the neck, back and the spine are relaxed along with mental relaxation which help in overcoming sleep problems.

iii) Pressure vibration

This is done with the fingertips in the downward direction of the vertebral column at the points of exit of the spinal nerves. The movement is one of shaking of the tissues and muscles by the flexion and extension of wrist joint or with the fingers from the meta carpo-phalangeal joints.

This movement has a soothing effect on the peripheral nerves and the central nervous system. The cells including the nerve cells are readily activated by this procedure.

Medicated oils

For treatment of sleep disorders massage may be done using almond oil, olive oil, mustard oil, sandalwood oil, coconut oil or pure "desi" ghee. These may be either massaged on the scalp, forehead, neck, back legs or sole of the feet before going to sleep. Medicated oils containing Brahmi (Harpestis miniera) bala, amruta, ashwagandha, shatavari, gotu kola, Bhringaraj and Mandukparni have a cooling effect on the mind. Aromatic essential oils like lotus, rose, mogra, lemon grass, khus, blue camomile, clary sage, laudanum, rose gardenia, jasmine and lavender are also very useful in treating sleep disorders. Mahanarayan oil is used to remove stiffness in the muscles and joints especially the neck muscles, scalp and forehead.

6. Ayurvedic Remedies in Sleep Disorders

Ayurveda is the ancient science of health and healing based on the principles of Atharvaveda. The fundamental principles of Ayurveda are based on "Dasha-Dhatu-Mala-Vijnana, *i.e.* the triad of the body elements responsible for the sustenance of the living body in their normal state and disease or ill-health when they are in the abnormal state.

1. "Brahmi" is a very effective medication used in the treatment of sleep disorders. It may be given alone in the form of juice or along with honey or the powdered bark of "Kulanjana" (Alpine galanga). "Brahmi Tel" is also very soothing when massaged on the head. "Brahmi ghrita" is also very effective when taken in the dose of 30-50 gm with milk.
2. Nutmeg of Jaiphal is another useful Ayurvedic preparation. When powdered and mixed with ghee and applied on the forehead or eyelids it can induce sleep effectively. The powder of nutmeg in the dose of 30 to 50 gm taken orally is also effective.
3. "Ashwagandha churna" in the dose of 20-30 gm with sugar and ghee is a very good remedy for insomnia. Also Ashwagandharishta taken in the dose of two teaspoonful after meals is very effective in inducing sleep.
4. The mucilage prepared by infusing two parts of the poppy seeds ("Ramadana") and one part of lettuce seeds ("Kahu") in water taken with sugar is very effective.
5. "Nidrodaya Rasa" in the dose of 15-20 gm with honey is a powerful hypnotic agent.
6. About 25-50 gm of "Chandravabha" with milk twice a day is another useful remedy for sleep disorders.
7. "Saraswata Churna" in the dose of 20 to 30 gm with honey is a very good medicine for treating insomnia. "Saraswatarishta" in the dose of two teaspoonfuls after meals has a soothing effect on the nervous system.
8. For people with problems of sleepwalking "Krimi Mudgar Rasa" along with "Vatakulantaka Rasa" in the dose of 125 mg with milk is a very effective remedy.
9. "Praval Panchamrat Rasa" in the dose of 250 to 500 mg along with ghee and "Sitopaladi Churna" one to two gm can induce an early sleep.

10. Certain patent medicines available for treating sleep disorders are: Calmtone, Bravobol and Relief and tablets Sunidra, Traquinyl, Siledin, Brain, Smritika, Yogini, Nidrayani and Nidrakarak and syrup Braintone.

Home remedies

1. Take half-teaspoonful of green coriander ("dhaniya") and add some sugar grains or honey and swallow it.
2. Before going to sleep one glassful of mango juice mixed with some milk should be drunk.
3. Boil a few grains of aniseed ("saunf") in water and drink it to get a sound sleep.
4. A small piece of dried and mashed ginger boiled in water until a concentrated solution is obtained should be taken before sleep.
5. A cup of juice of papaya is also useful.
6. Apple jelly or mashed apple should be eaten before sleep.
7. To a cup of curd add a few grams of sugar, aniseed and powdered black pepper and consumed in the evening.
8. To half a teaspoonful of lemon juice add one teaspoonful of honey and swallow.
9. Fresh goat's milk and mustard oil mixed with camphor should be massaged on the feet to get a good sleep.
10. To one glass of warm milk add some honey or one teaspoonful of ghee and drink it just before going to bed.
11. A medium-size onion should be well-fried in ghee and eaten to get a sound sleep.
12. If fresh flowers of henna plant ("Mehndi") are kept on the pillow, they can induce sleep.
13. Saffron should be fried in ghee and the vapours inhaled.

7. Magnetotherapy

Definition

Magnetotherapy is a branch of medicine in which human diseases are treated by the application of magnets to the body of the patients. It is the simplest, cheapest and painless system of medicine with absolutely no side effects.

Dr. E.K. Maclean of New York has successfully treated advanced cases of cancer with an electromagnetic activator. He has claimed that cancer cannot exist in a strong magnetic field.

Treatment of sleep disorders by magnetotherapy

1. The South Pole of a low power crescent ceramic magnet may be kept on the forehead between the eyebrows for 10 to 15 minutes before going to sleep for a week or ten days. This will induce a sound sleep for many months.
2. In case the above magnet is ineffective in a week's time, a medium-power cast alloy magnet may be applied at the same place for 5 to 10 minutes every night.

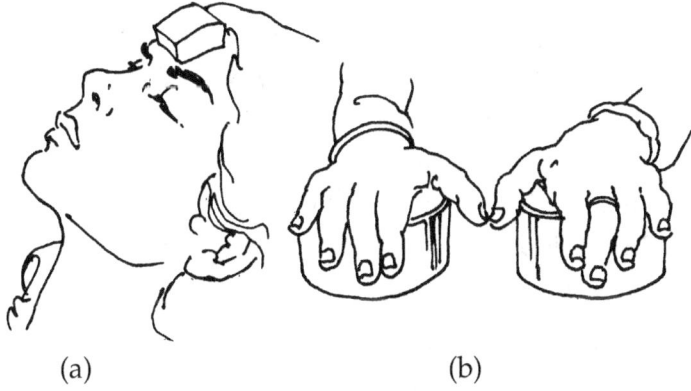

(a)   (b)

Fig 28 (a): South Pole of Magnet on Forehead
(b): North Pole under palm of right hand

3. If both these magnets are not effective in inducing sleep, a high-powered cast alloy magnet may be applied under both the palms.
4. Simultaneously, water magnetised with South Pole in the dose of two to three ounces 3-4 times daily for adults and smaller doses for children is also very useful for treating sleep disorders.
5. A magnetic head belt worn on forehead for 15 to 30 minutes once or twice a day for a week or ten days is another useful technique for curing insomnia. This is very effective in patients who have disturbed sleep due to neurological or psychiatric disorders.

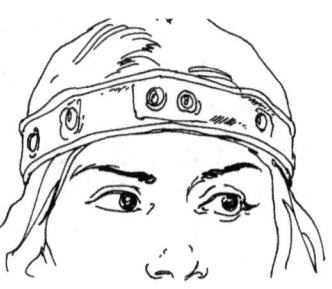

Fig 29: Magnetic Head Belt

Adverse effects

Sometimes adverse effects are seen in those using high powered electromagnets:

1. Mild tingling sensation in hands and feet
2. A feeling of warmth in the body
3. Heaviness of head
4. Dryness of tongue
5. Increased urge for urination
6. Mild giddiness
7. Sweating in the areas on contact with magnets

Precautions

❑ The ideal time is in the morning, preferably on empty stomach and after a bath.
❑ Avoid eating or drinking cold things for at least one hour after applying high-power magnets.

- ❏ Since magnetotherapy produces some heat in the body, bath should be avoided for at least one hour after treatment.
- ❏ If high or medium-powered magnets are applied after full meals, they may cause nausea.
- ❏ High-power magnets should not be applied to pregnant women, very weak people and to children.
- ❏ High-power magnets should not be applied directly to delicate organs of the body namely eyes, head and heart.
- ❏ Watches should not be allowed to come in contact with magnets unless they are anti-magnetic.
- ❏ When high-power magnets are applied for long periods they may produce heaviness in head, giddiness, yawning, tingling in nerves etc. Discontinue contact with magnets and rest immediately.
- ❏ Opposite poles of high-power magnets should not be brought near each other face to face as they attract each other with great force.
- ❏ When high-power or medium-power magnets are not in use they should be kept joined with a keeper so that their magnetism is not wasted and they are not demagnetised soon.
- ❏ When taking magnetic treatment under palms, it is not necessary to remove gold or silver rings from the finger.

8. Acupressure & Reflexology

It is believed that in our body there is presence of bioenergy or bioelectrical activity which makes us move, breathe, eat and even think. This energy is called Prana or Chetana in India while Chinese call it chi which consists of Yin or negative force and Ÿang or positive force. These forces or bioenergy flow through definite channels in the body called meridians or Jing.

There are 14 meridians in our body of which 12 are located in pairs on either side of the body while the remaining two are single and lay on the front and back of the body. The 12 paired meridians comprise six Yin meridians starting from the toes or mid-part of the body and reaching the head or fingers and six Ÿang meridians in the reverse direction.

These meridians maintain the flow of bioelectricity and are connected with the main organs or systems of the body. One end of each meridian lies in the hand, the leg or the face and the other in the main organ after which it is named. This is the reason why pressure applied to a particular point in the hand or the leg affects the remote organ connected with this point.

The 14 meridians are as follows:

1. Large intestine meridian
2. Stomach meridian
3. Small intestine meridian
4. Bladder intestine meridian
5. Triple warmer meridian
6. Gall bladder meridian
7. Lung meridian
8. Spleen meridian
9. Kidney meridian
10. Heart meridian
11. Heart constrictor or Pericardium meridian
12. Liver meridian
13. Governing vessel meridian
14. Conception vessel meridian

Each of the 14 main meridians has subsidiary meridians. If the flow of bioenergy in a meridian is not proper, it can be corrected by stimulating certain points on the meridian by applying pressure on them. Thus the disease of that organ can be eliminated and the pain in these points is relieved as soon as the disease is eliminated.

Pain at any point on the body is possibly a symptom of some disorder in an organ or in a system of the body. If pressure is methodically applied to this point, the disease or disorder can be removed.

Effects of acupressure

1. It reduces pain of different types, *e.g.* joint pain, headache, backache, toothache, sprains etc.
2. It also has a tranquillising or sedative effect on the brain. If an EEG is done while doing acupressure, it shows depression of delta & theta waves.
3. It strengthens the body's natural resistance power due to which the respiratory rate, heartbeat, blood pressure, body temperature and metabolism becomes normal. There is also increase in the red and white blood cells and gamma globulins, and cholesterol and triglycerides are decreased.
4. Depression, anxiety, stress and tension are controlled with acupressure due to its effect on the brain.
5. Muscles and joints are strengthened by acupressure and are useful in treatment of polio, paralysis and other neuromuscular disorders.

Reflexology or zone therapy

Reflexology refers to the form of treatment which involves giving a massage to certain reflex areas of the feet and hands.

The body is divided into 10 longitudinal zones. If a straight line is drawn through the centre of the body, the whole body is divided into five zones on either side of the body. Zone one extends from the thumb, up the arm to the brain and then down to the big toe; and zone two extends from second finger, up the arm to the brain and down to the third toe. Similarly the other zones of equal width occur through the body from front to back. They are like segments of the body and not fine lines like acupuncture meridian lines. The line marking between each zone extends from the web of finger to the web of the toe. Whichever parts of the body are found within a certain zone, these parts are linked to one another by energy flow within the zone and can therefore affect one another. Treatment is done by applying pressure to accessible areas within the same zone. Pressure is applied using cloth pegs, metal combs, elastic bands or metal probes around the hands and fingers as well as toes, ankles, wrists, elbows or knees. The amount of pressure applied should be between one and 10 kg for an interval of 30 seconds to 5 minutes.

The reflex areas of the feet and hands are divided into transverse zones. Zone one refers to all parts of the body above the shoulder girdle, while zone two refers to those parts between the shoulder girdle and waist. Zone three refers to organs below the waist.

Technique of reflexology
The thumb is held bent and the side and end of the thumb is pressed into the part of the foot or hand to be treated. The other fingers of the hand will rest gently round the foot. Certain meridians are present in the sole of feet and their massage in the direction of flow of energy stimulates the organ. Massaging in the opposite direction gives a soothing effect.

Advantages of acupressure
1. It is an easy, simple, reflective form of the treatment.
2. It can be done in the privacy of one's own house.
3. Treatment can be done anytime of the day.
4. No money is to be spent to get benefits of treatment.
5. No side-effects are observed with this treatment.
6. In this form of treatment the person looks after his own health.

7. In some cases, acupressure can be used as a first aid measure till the doctor arrives or if the patient is admitted to the hospital.
8. It helps prevent relapses of the diseases.
9. It associates with other forms of treatment. It gives a speedy relief.
10. It increases the efficiency of the organs and systems of body and strengthens joints and muscles.
11. Even in serious diseases it prevents aggravation of symptoms.
12. It establishes the convention of touch communication or touch healing and establishes rapport between doctor and patient.

Acupressure points in insomnia

Today we come across a number of persons suffering from insomnia. They get to sleep only for an hour or two or something likewise. They toss in their beds for the whole night. According to the figures available, millions of rupees are spent every year on sleeping pills; but these drugs have two risks: (1) They produce side-effects. (2) People gradually become addicted to them. Compared to such drugs, acupressure is a safe and more effective remedy.

Acupressure points: (1) The point located on the forehead between the two eyebrows. (2) The point located in the depression behind the lobe of the ear. (3) The point located on the fleshy part between the thumb and the index finger. (4) The point located on the base of the palm in line with the little finger. (5) The point slightly behind and four finger breadths above the inner prominence of the ankle bone. (6) The point located below the inner prominence of the ankle bone. (7) The point located under the outer prominence of the ankle bone. (8) The points located on the ear as shown in the figure.

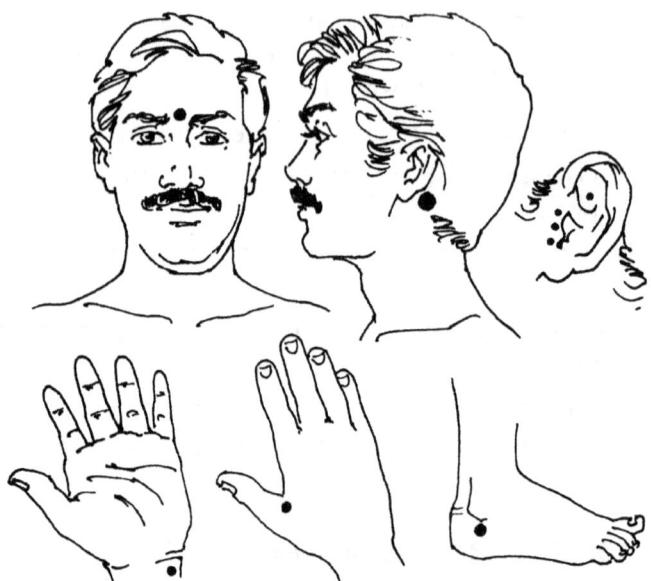

Fig 30: Acupressure Points in Insomnia

Treatment : Take acupressure treatment three or four times a day. Treatment may also be taken alternately on the first four points and the remaining four points. It is necessary to take this treatment before going to bed. Take treatment on each point for two to four minutes.

9. Chromotherapy

Chromotherapy refers to treatment of diseases using colours. This is usually done in the following manner :-

1. Direct radiation to the affected part/organ of the body.
2. Application of oils, ghee, glycerine etc. charged with specific colour to the affected part.
3. Drinking water irradiated in specific coloured bottles.
4. Using medicines charged with specific colours.
5. Eating specific coloured food items.
6. Inhaling gases charged in coloured containers.

7. Wearing clothes of specific colours.
8. Living/sleeping in a room painted with the specific colours.

Use of chromotherapy in sleep disorders

Direct radiation

Blue colour is best suited for treatment of sleep disorders.

Take a table lamp and attach it with either blue coloured bulb or cover the existing bulb with blue coloured cellophane paper. Apply the direct rays of light from this lamp to the scalp, forehead and back of neck for up to 10-15 minutes daily. This should be ideally done at night for an hour or throughout the night.

Keeping a blue zero watt bulb on, during the night in the bedroom, can also help in giving direct radiations to the whole body.

Local application of irradiated oils, ghee etc.

Take a blue coloured bottle or a white bottle covered with blue cellophane paper. Fill it with coconut oil or mustard oil or olive oil or ghee and place it on a dry wooden board exposed to the direct sunlight. It should be exposed for about 45 days. It should be kept in sunlight during the day and kept in a safe place at night. In case of non-availability of natural light, artificial light may be used as a substitute. The bottles should be dusted daily. Such colour charged oils can be stored for months or even one to two years.

This irradiated oil or ghee can be used to massage the scalp, forehead and neck to give excellent results to people suffering from insomnia and other sleep disorders.

Drinking irradiated water

Using the procedure given above, water can be charged in blue-coloured bottles. This should be charged in direct sunlight for as many days as possible. This should be drunk in the dose of one cup early in the morning and half a cup before lunch and dinner.

Eating specific coloured food items

Since blue and violet colours soothe the mind and help in cases of sleep disorders, consuming fruits and vegetables of such colours can be useful.

The fruits and vegetables of such colours are blue plums, blue berries, black berries, blue grapes, purple grapes, phalsa, jamun, eggplant, purple broccoli, beet tops, black carrots, kanji of black carrots, viola odorata (banafsha) etc.

Clothing

Wearing blue or violet coloured clothes can prove to be very useful for people who have problems with sleep. Wearing a blue or violet coloured night-suit and sleeping on a bed with bed sheet, pillows and bed covers of blue colour can give rise to an undisturbed sleep at night.

Colour scheme in the bedroom

If the bedroom walls are painted with blue enamel paint and the furniture and other items are of the same colour in the bedroom, it can create wonders. If such individuals wear blue night-dress and have the same colour combination with bedding, lighting etc., there can be no problem in attaining sound sleep.

10. Music Therapy

It is a form of treatment using music and musical instruments in order to restore, maintain and improve physical, physiological, psychological and spiritual health and well-being.

Application of music therapy

Music therapy has been found to be useful in various diseases. They are as follows:

a. Sleep disorders

By virtue of its relaxing effect on the mind, music therapy has benefited patients of insomnia to the maximum extent. People who have difficulty either in the initiation of sleep or its maintenance as well as those with nightmares, night terrors, sleepwalking or even heavy sleepers have benefited from it.

b. Dementia and Alzheimer's disease

Elderly individuals with organic (degenerative) diseases such as, memory problems, poor sleep, abnormal behaviour and speech problems improve considerably with this form of treatment.

c. Depression

Patients with depression who are often sad, socially withdrawn and unable to cope at home and office often find solace in music. If "Raga Darbari Kanada" is practiced regularly by such individuals they will not require any antidepressant medications.

d. Anxiety neurosis

People who are always tense, excited, worried, stressed and disturbed sleep, often enjoy the benefits of music. "Raga Gorakh Kalyan" has helped many people in overcoming stress and tension.

e. Schizophrenia

This is a dreaded mental illness characterised by social withdrawal, suspiciousness, abnormal behaviour, hallucinations and sleep problems. Music has a soothing effect on such individuals; encouraging them for social interactions, better physical, mental and emotional activity and sound sleep.

f. Acute and chronic pain

Music therapy acts as a painkiller in individuals with severe chronic pain. Many dentists and surgeons have reduced the dose of anesthesia while performing minor surgeries in patients by just playing soothing music for such individuals. Pain due to arthritis, toothache, abdominal colic, headache etc. can also be similarly controlled. Thus music can play the role of an anesthetic agent.

g. Hypertension

People with hypertension (high blood pressure) along with a headache and sleep problems often stop taking medicines when they tune to the music and also start singing and playing musical instruments. Daily recitation or humming of "Bhairava Raga" before sunrise can control heart disease.

h. Stroke

Patients with stroke who have weakness on one side or one half of the body with memory and speech problem improve when a favourite melody is played to them. If they attempt singing and dancing the results are miraculous.

i. Stuttering and speech disorders

Individuals with stuttering or stammering and other speech disorders can often sing well without any difficulty though speaking a sentence may be difficult for them. When these people start singing regularly their speech problems are often cured.

j. Hyperactive children

Hyperactive children with irritability, inattentiveness, abnormal behaviour, lack of muscular coordination and poor performance in school benefit from music therapy.

k. Mentally-retarded children

Children who are mentally-retarded and have difficulty in movements of the body, speech, memory and coordination improve with music therapy.

l. Polio

Patients of polio who have difficulty in walking improve considerably with music therapy.

m. Pregnancy

Researchers have shown that if the music is regularly heard by pregnant women, the growth of the body is normal and delivery is easier. Moreover the type of music also affects the mental make-up of the children when they grow up.

n. Tinnitus

Tinnitus is a disease of the inner part of the ear and brain which is characterised by ringing, humming and hissing sounds or noises in the ears. E.N.T surgeons recommend music therapy to mask these noises in the ears.

o. Substance abuse or drug addiction

Patients of drug addiction or substance abuse have been found to give up their habit when their treatment is supplemented with music.

p. Head injury

Patients with head injury are found to respond favourably to music therapy with early improvement in their neurological symptoms/deficit.

q. Terminally-ill patients

If proper "ragas" are used even the terminally-ill patients can be successfully treated. It is reported that St. Tyagaraj, a south Indian musician saint brought a person back to life by singing "Raga Bilhari."

How music therapy helps patients of sleep disorders?

When music therapy is used in sleep disorders, the following beneficial changes are observed:

1. Complete relaxation of the muscles of the body is observed.
2. Mental stress and tension, which are a major factors in sleep problems are controlled.
3. There is a vast improvement in mood and behaviour of the individual.
4. There is an increased sense of well-being of the person who listens to music.
5. Pain in the body, if any, is controlled.
6. The heartbeat and blood pressure is reduced, which is useful for the patients with insomnia.
7. There is improvement in the cardiac output or blood circulation which invigorates the whole body.
8. The immune system is boosted up which combats various diseases in the body.

11. Aromatherapy

Aromatherapy refers to the application of certain aromatic/scented oils as a form of treatment for many disorders.

Methods of aromatherapy

Methods of applying these fragrant, precious oils are given below:

a. Inhalation

Add a few drops of essential oil to a bowl of boiling water. A towel is placed over the head and the scented vapours are inhaled. This method is very useful for patients with diseases of the respiratory system.

b. Diffusion

Spray a few drops of fragrant oil in the air in a closed room. This method is useful for enhancing the freshness in the room, keeping the nerves calm, producing a sense of well-being and improving respiratory illnesses.

c. Massage

Certain aromatic oils may be rubbed on the skin to produce results. Most relaxant creams contain aromatic oils for treating muscular sprain, pain and stiffness of joints.

d. Bathing

A few drops of oil can be added to a tub full of water or a Jacuzzi and a bath taken. Alternately a wet sponge or cloth is dipped in oil and kept on the body and a shower bath is taken.

e. Hot and cold compresses

A few drops of oil are added to hot and cold water alternately and applied to areas of pain, aches or bruises.

f. Other techniques

These include applying a few drops on a pillow or clothes or shoe rack, heating the oil in a ring burner or sprinkling the oils over the burning logs of wood during a "havana" or in the fireplace.

The aromatic oils useful in sleep disorders

1. Lavender
2. Peppermint
3. Rosemary
4. Chamomile
5. Tarragon
6. Neroli
7. Ylang-Ylang

These oils help in relaxing the body and triggering off soothing effects in the brain. They also reduce stress, relieve anxiety, remove stiffness in the body and improve the sense of overall well-being.

Contraindications of aromatherapy

Aromatherapy should be avoided in the following conditions.

Bronchial asthma – Some essential oils can trigger off bronchial spasms. Hence, if one is suffering from or is prone to develop bronchial asthma, he should avoid aromatherapy.

Skin allergy – Some people are allergic towards many oral and skin allergens. They should not use these oils in their bath. To find out if he is allergic to a particular oil, he should place one drop of oil on his forearm and observe for 24 hours for any untoward reactions.

Pregnancy – It is better to avoid aromatherapy especially rosemary, sage and juniper oils during pregnancy. These oils are known to cause uterine contractions when taken in excessive amounts.

Infants and children – Aromatherapy should be avoided in infants and children especially on their face. Also peppermint oil should not be used in children less than 3 years.

Adverse effects

Internal application

Since essential oils are highly concentrated, taking them internally or orally can lead to toxic effects in the body. Therefore, they should not be ingested without the doctor's approval.

Skin allergy

Except lavender no other concentrated oil should be used on the skin.

Effect on eyes

These oils should be kept away from the eyes even while applying on the body or inhaling. Some oils can also cause sunburns due to their heightened sensitivity to sunlight.

Headache & fatigue

Excessive inhalation of vapours of essential oils can cause headache and fatigue.

12. Feng Shui and its Role in Sleep Disorders

What is Feng Shui?

Feng Shui is the ancient Chinese art of living in harmony with the environment. It uses "Chi" (energy) to determine the positive and negative aspects of a home, office, building or factory environment.

Basic philosophy

It is based on the theory that there is an invisible energy that flows through the universe, through our body, the food we eat, our home and workplace and the environment around us. It is known as "Prana" in India "Chi" in China and "Ki" in Japan.

According to a map or "Bagua" living spaces are divided into nine areas – career, knowledge, health, wealth, fame, relationships, children, travel and good luck. Energising of these respective areas can enhance these qualities or areas of life.

How it works?

It mainly works through colour schemes, placement of furniture, lighting, plants and reflective objects such as sculptures, paintings and art. To produce proper impact they should be so arranged that they are harmonious with the forces of nature or cosmic energy. Hence, one can improve one's health, wealth, relationship, knowledge, career etc.

Feng Shui measures for treating sleep-related problems

- The bedroom should be ideally located in the South-west portion of the house known as the area for marriage and romantic happiness.
- If it is not possible to allocate the bedroom in this area, the bed should be so aligned that the head points preferably towards the South-west or South. This allows the "Chi" energy to flow into the body while sleeping.
- The head or the feet should not point towards the door while sleeping since these are known as "coffin positions."
- If there is an attached toilet or bathroom in the bedroom, the occupants should not face the entrance in this room because they will breathe in negative "Chi" throughout the night.
- If the long side of the bed is against the same wall as the entrance, one should not sleep with his back to the wall.
- The bed should not be lying under an exposed beam on the ceiling. In case there is no alternative, the bed should be placed in such a way that the beam runs parallel to the bed and not across it. As a remedy, two bamboo flutes can be hung from the beam tied with red thread or ribbon.
- The bedroom should receive sufficient light during the forenoon while the curtains may be drawn in the afternoon and night.
- The dressing table should face South-west but never the foot end of the bed.
- The bathroom and toilet should not be in the northern side of the house. If present, avoid using it or keep the lid down and the door closed. A large mirror

- may also be placed outside its door to symbolically make it disappear.
- ❑ Never keep anything related to the office or do office work in the bedroom.
- ❑ Keep metallic wind chimes with hollow rods in the bedroom, which help in the flow of beneficial "Chi" flowing through the home whenever they move. Alternately hanging a crystal can provide positive energy and banish nightmares.
- ❑ Blue or violet coloured lights and blue or violet painting of the bedroom walls create a relaxed atmosphere in the room conducive for a sound sleep. Burning a small blue or violet candle in the bedroom every evening is also useful.
- ❑ The bedroom should be free of all clutter or useless things, which impede the free flow of energy into the bedroom.
- ❑ All electrical appliances in the bedroom should be unplugged or switched off at night or persons should sleep at least 4 feet away from these appliances. This is to avoid man-made electromagnetic fields or radiations.
- ❑ Keeping hibiscus in the bedroom promotes sexual compatibility. Jasmine is considered to be an aphrodisiac and anti-depressant. The Tulsi plant helps in keeping away evil thoughts and arresting the negative energy of any visitor into the house.
- ❑ The atmosphere can be energised by regular burning of incense or performing "havan".

13. Medical Treatment—A Critical Analysis

Medical treatment of sleep disorders does not usually mean just taking some sleeping pills. It involves a detailed history of the problem and identifying the cause of the disorder.

Medicines commonly used in the treatment of sleep disorders

These may be classified as follow:-

Hypnotics

Hypnotics are the agents which have the exclusive property of inducing sleep. The examples of medicines in this group are the barbiturates like phenobarbitone (*Gardenal, Luminal*) amylobarbitone, pentobarbitone and thiopentone. Other hypnotics are chloral hydrate, clichbraphenazone, triclofos and methaqualone.

Hypnotics are used only in cases of severe intractable sleep disorders. Their usage is also limited due to their toxicity effects, withdrawal symptoms and liability to abuse.

Sedatives and tranquilisers

These groups of medicines are very commonly used to the extent of being misused. Examples of sedatives are diazepam (Calmpose, Valium, Paxum, Placidox), alprazolam (Alprax, Anxit, Trika, Zoldac, Restyl) Ativan, Larpose, Librium, Equilibrium, Nindral, Lyzop, Nitravet, Hypnptex etc.

These medicines help in treating sleep disorders as well as control symptoms of anxiety and depression which may be sometimes the underlying causes of sleep problems.

Anti-depressants and anti-psychotic agents

In some individuals with sleep disorders, who have an underlying mental illness, these medicines are used. Popular brands of these medicines are Depsonil, Antidep, Surmontil, Tryptomer, Clofranil, Demelox, Lozapin, Fludac, Prothiaden, Serenace, Halidol, Orap, Respidon, Thioril, Trinicalm, Flumap etc.

Adverse/side-effects of these medicines

Certain side-effects have been observed with the medicines given in the table below.

1. Daytime drowsiness
2. Headache
3. Giddiness
4. Confusion
5. Forgetfulness
6. Disturbance in the digestive system
7. Fall in blood pressure
8. Skin rashes, itching
9. Blurred vision, double vision
10. Change in libido (sex drive)
11. Drug dependence and withdrawal symptoms
12. Slurred speech
13. Poor appetite
14. Feeling of weakness, lethargy
15. Lack of inhibitions
16. Poor concentration
17. Tolerance to drugs or habituation
18. Not safe in pregnant and breastfeeding women and men above 60 years
19. Sexual dysfunction, *e.g.* erectile disturbance and ejaculatory problems
20. Cleft palate (a deformity in mouth), reported in the newborn
21. May worsen certain mental disease, *e.g.* Parkinsonism, mania

Conditions in which medicines are useful

There are certain conditions in which medicines may be given but only for a few days or up to two weeks. In cases of emergency intermittent treatment for up to three to four weeks may be given. Conditions in which medicines are beneficial are given in the table below:-

Conditions in which medicines are beneficial

1. Sleep disorders associated with
   a) Mental illness
   b) Behavioural problems
   c) Drug abuse
   d) Alcohol withdrawal
   e) Emotional problem—death of a beloved, rape, kidnapping etc.
   f) Physical illness
2. Panic disorders
3. Phobias
4. Night terrors/nightmares
5. Sleepwalking

Points to remember

1. Sedatives and tranquillisers increase daytime drowsiness which aggravates insomnia at night.
2. Prolonged usage of these agents can produce short form memory impairment.
3. Daytime alertness, concentration and muscular coordination may be reduced.
4. In tolerance to drugs increases and higher dosages are required to produce sleep.
5. Sleeping pills should not be consumed before or after an alcoholic drink.
6. All option for treatment of insomnia should be tried before resorting to drugs.

14. Other General Tips

Certain general tips or rules should be followed in order to get good sound sleep at night. These are given below:

Do's	Don'ts
1. Go to bed every night at a fixed time.	1. Don't attend late night parties, movies and discos etc.
2. Sleep early and wake up early.	2. Don't read horror stories, violent adventure stories or sexually exciting literature before going to sleep.
3. Have a sleep for atleast 6-8 hours.	3. Don't see horror movies/programmes depicting sex, crime, and violence before bed time.
4. Sleep in a well-ventilated room on a cosy and firm bed.	4. Don't listen to high voltage pop or western music before bed time.
5. Sleep on your back.	5. Don't drink tea, coffee or alcohol before going to sleep.
6. Eat a light dinner non-spicy, non-oily and easily digestible.	6. Don't eat a heavy, spicy and oily dinner.
7. Have dinner 2-3 hours before sleeping.	7. Don't go to sleep immediately after dinner.
8. Take a small stroll if possible after dinner.	8. Don't take sleeping pills or alcohol or smoke to induce sleep.
9. Drink a glass of hot milk before going to sleep.	9. Avoid zarda, gutka, tobacco, khaini, pan masala or alcohol.
10. A warm water bath or an oil massage before sleep is very useful.	10. Don't have illuminated or musical clocks in the bedroom.
11. Mask sounds and noises in the bedroom with a fan or A.C. or by tuning in to static F.M.	11. Don't sleep in the afternoon except for a short nap.

Do's	Don'ts
12. Sex at bedtime is the natural sedative for relaxing the body and mind.	12. Don't think negatively about life and daily events.
13. Read a religious book or listen to soft music or watch light movies/programmes before going to sleep.	
14. Recite Gayatri Mantra or a prayer or meditate just before going to sleep.	
15. For tensions of office work write down the problems and try to solve them before going to sleep.	
16. Backward counting while lying in bed is also useful.	
17. A positive attitude towards life can help in overcoming stress and anxiety.	

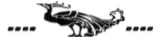

Chapter 11

Lifestyle Suggestions To Enhance Sleep

Sleep is an important constituent of our life. In case you are not getting adequate sleep you would feel irritable at the workplace, gain weight, develop thyroid problems and suffer lack of concentration. You would be open to many allergies, tissue breakdown inappropriate aggression, indigestion, pain in joints and knee. All these adverse affects make you stressful and disturb your peace of mind. The negative aspects of inadequate sleep can be overcome by the undermentioned lifestyle suggestions that enhance your sleep.

- ❑ Set a sleep schedule making it part of a natural habit on all days of the year.
- ❑ Reduce or avoid as many drugs as possible.
- ❑ Consume alcohol in moderation if you are a regular drinker Alcohol initially helps you to get sleep but, in fact, it spoils your sleep pattern. Cut down on stimulants like excessive tea or coffee. A study shows that the caffeine is not metabolised efficiently. So an afternoon cup of coffee or tea even will keep some people from falling asleep at night.
- ❑ Drink chamormile or jasmine tea which does not contain caffeine and really refresh you.

- ❑ Eat a light dinner preferably two hours before sleeping.
- ❑ Drink a glass of warm milk before going to bed. It contains sleep inducing substance and simultaneously acts as a laxative for the morning stimulation.
- ❑ Avoid constipation of pan masala or tobacco.
- ❑ Try not to pick an argument before going to sleep.
- ❑ Don't read horror books or disturbing material at night.
- ❑ Avoid sleeping during the day.
- ❑ Switch off TV, laptop and smart phones an hour before going to bed. In fact, you should avoid watching TV in the bedroom.
- ❑ Make a regular habit of exercising for at least half an hour. Exercising in the morning is the best.
- ❑ Shed excess weight. Being overweight can disturb your sleep.
- ❑ Avoid sensitive foods such as too much of sweets and pasteurized products that cause excess congestion, gastrointestinal upset and other problems.
- ❑ If you are menopausal or perimonopausaul, get examined. The hormonal changes at this stage can may cause sleep problems.
- ❑ Increase your melatonin which can be done with exposure to bright sunlight. Melatonin is a natural substance made by your body enhancing sleep besides other several benefits.
- ❑ Sleep in absolute complete darkness or as close to it as possible because even the tiniest of light glowing from your clock could be interfering with your sleep. It also helps to decrease your risk of cancer.
- ❑ The temperature of your bedroom should be between 60 to 70°F.
- ❑ Check your bedroom for electromagnetic fields emitted from electrical and electronic gadgets. The

electromagnetic fields disrupt your pineal gland, production of melatonin and hormones that disturb your sleep. Some experts even recommend the switching of the entire power supply of your house.

- Avoid using loud alarm clock as the same is very stressful on your body to be suddenly jolted awake.
- Reserve your bed for sleeping only. Avoid watching TV on your bed or doing any paperwork. This way you may find if harder to relax and therefore, sleep.
- Consider having separate bedrooms if possible. Many people sharing a bed with a partner do not get proper sleep.
- Go to bed as early as possible. Your body does the majority of its recharging between 11 pm and 1 am.
- Don't drink too much fluids within two hours of going to bed.
- Go to the bathroom right before bed.
- If possible eat a high protein snack couple of hours before going to bed. It increases production of melatonin and serotonin which induce me sleep.
- Take a hot bath before going to bed. It is very effective in getting good sleep
- Wear socks to bed or you could place a hot water bottle near your feet at night. Feet often feel cold as compared to the rest of body.
- Put your work away at least one hour before going to bed giving your mind a chance to unwind soon. You can go to sleep feeling calm leaving behind worries of tomorrow.
- Listen to soothing music. Some people feel sound of ocean or forest to be shooting for sleep .
- Do alternate nostril breathing while listening to soothing music.
- Try to learn and do the progressive relaxation exercises to relax all parts of the body.

- ❏ Meditate for some time to release the negative emotions.
- ❏ Chant any mantra depending on your faith
- ❏ Read a spiritual book before going to bed
- ❏ Chamomile, lavender, tagora and valerian are very useful sedative herbs for insomnia.
- ❏ Auto-suggestions are also very effective for a sound sleep. You can advise or command yourself to sleep.
- ❏ Self hypnosis can also be done for making your body tension free.

Chapter 12

Recent Advances in Diagnosis Treatment of Sleep Disorders

With advancement in science and technology, there has been immense progress in the diagnosis and treatment modalities of different diseases. So is the case of sleep disorders where better facilities have developed for their diagnosis and treatment.

Sleep Medicine

A new branch of sleep medicine has been added recently to the medical curriculum. It deals with minute details about the types of sleep disorders, their clinical features, complications, modes of diagnosis, prevention and treatment. Doctors who complete this course are referred to as Sleep Specialists/Physicians.

Sleep Laboratories

In order to diagnose sleep disorders, the history alone is not sufficient. Certain tests are done in specialised diagnostics centres under the guidance of sleep specialists. These centres contain sophisticated instruments and the patient has to stay here overnight and undergo certain tests. These centres are known as Sleep Laboratories.

Sleep Clinics

In many major hospitals and referred centres, a sleep clinic/O.P.D. is available for the diagnosis of sleep disorders. Such clinics are manned by a team of sleep specialists along with physicians, E.N.T. specialists, neurologist and psychiatrists. These clinics help in the proper diagnosis and treatment of sleep disorders.

Utility of sleep clinics & laboratories

Sleep Clinics and Sleep Laboratories have the following advantages:-

1. They are very useful in diagnosing different types of sleep disorders.
2. Medical conditions which occur during sleep can be accurately detected and treated.
3. Normal sleeping patterns can be restored in those with sleep disorders.
4. Newer treatment modalities can be tried.
5. Preventive aspects of sleep disorders can be highlighted by sleep physicians.
6. A collaborative study of sleep disorders can be done under one roof.

Sleep Hygiene

This is a new term which refers to general advice that may help to promote a good sleep pattern. This includes the environment in the bedroom, timing of exercise, dietary advice and Do's and Don'ts pertaining to lifestyle.

Diseases Occurring During Sleep

Many diseases are present or deteriorate only during sleep and are usually adequately compensated for during the day. Sleep Medicines and Sleep Laboratories have expanded the knowledge regarding these diseases. Angina pain is more likely to occur during the N.R.E.M phase of sleep. Breathlessness while sleeping may indicate the presence of severe bronchial asthma or heart diseases. Pain of peptic ulcer is more severe at night due to increased production of acid in the stomach. Similarly, reflux esophagitis with the backward flow of acid into the mouth occurs at night. Cluster headache is reported in the early morning hours. Snoring is believed to be related to hypertension and heart disease in many individuals.

Innovative Diagnostic Technologies

Due to development advancement in Sleep Medicine newer diagnostic tools have been developed. These can be used to accurately diagnose the sleep disorders by Sleep Physicians in the Sleep Laboratories.

Some of the important diagnostic tests used to diagnose sleep disorders are given below:-

Sleep Studies/Polysomnography/ Rapid Eye Movement Studies

This is a test of sleep cycles and stages through the use of continuous recordings of brain waves (E.E.G.), electrical activities of muscles (electromyogram) eye movement (electro-oculogram) respiratory rate, blood pressure, blood oxygen saturation (oximetry) and heart rhythm (E.C.G.) and direct observation of the person during sleep and semi quantitative recording of muscles of chest and abdomen to evaluate breathing patterns.

Stages of Sleep

There are two stages of sleep – R.E.M or Rapid Eye Movement Sleep and N.R.E.M or Non-Rapid Eye Movement sleep. R.E.M. sleep is associated with dreaming and generalised muscle paralysis except the eye muscles and diaphragm. N.R.E.M sleep has four stages distinguishable by E.E.G. waves. R.E.M sleep alternates with N.R.E.M sleep approximately every 90 minutes. A person with normal sleep usually has 4 to 5 hours of R.E.M & N.R.E.M sleep at night.

Procedure

The test (polysomnogram) is conducted in a sleep study centre. It is carried out during the night so that normal sleep patterns can be reproduced. Electrodes are placed on the scalp, the outer edge of the eyelids and the skin on the chin in preparation for the test. Characteristic patterns from the electrodes are recorded during wakefulness with the eyes closed and during sleep. The time taken to fall asleep is measured as well as the time to enter R.E.M. sleep. Sometimes the movements of a person during sleep are recorded by video camera.

Indications for the test

The test is performed for insomnia, excessive daytime sleepiness, obstructive sleep apnea, breathing difficulties during sleep or behaviour-related disturbances during sleep.

Multiple Sleep Latency Test (M.S.L.T.)

This test is done in a quiet and dark room or in the sleep-laboratory. The patient is asked to try to fall asleep for about 20 minutes at two hourly intervals on 5 occasions during the day under ideal conditions for sleep. The time taken to go to sleep is noted. If the person falls asleep in less than 5 minutes on 3 or more occasions during the tests, he is diagnosed to suffer from excessive daytime sleepiness.

For reliable results the duration of sleep during the previous night should be known. Moreover, the patient must abstain from drugs, alcohol and coffee before the test.

Questionnaires & Symptoms Check-list

The diagnosis of sleep disorders is sometimes done on the basis of certain questionnaires which determine the disease or sleeping habits subjectively. Certain subjective scales are also available, *e.g.* Epworth Sleepiness Scale and Stanford Sleepiness Scale. Questionnaires based on symptoms can also decipher the sleep architecture, personality, mental status and the point at which the person wakes up or the type of sleep disorder.

Portable Sleep Studies
Recently, portable instruments have been designed in which the recordings of sleep studies or polysomnography can be done at home. Innovative technology can give rise to similar tests as done by the patient himself in the form of a video-cassette attached to his chest using HOLSTER for heart diseases.

Dreams and Medical Illness
Current research has shown that dreams may reflect the presence of cause or precipitate organic disease. It may serve as a marker for either psychological conflict or personality traits that might influence the development of organic diseases. Prospective studies have shown that among men dreams of death and among women dreams of separation, correlate with severe heart disease. Dreams of lost resources have been correlated with the finding of brain disease in elderly individuals. Changes in the amount, quality and difficulty in remembering dreams may reflect neurological damage.

Sleep Mattresses
Recently special mattresses, pillows and quilts have been designed which use the theory of magnetic forces and acupressure. They help in improving blood circulation, relieve back pain and constipation, reduce fatigue and give rise to sound sleep. It is claimed that the person using these devices feels energetic and fully charged on waking up in the morning.

Reiki
Reiki is a 200-year old Japanese healing technique which has of late come to the forefront.

It is based on the theory that all living beings have an energy system known as "Chi" and that blockage of this energy in the human body can lead to illness and disharmony. There are certain "chakras" or energy-centres which can be activated by regular meditation and "charging of these areas by touch-therapy". People who regularly practise meditation, especially involving the "chakras in the crown of the head and forehead", never suffer from insomnia.

Gadgets for sound sleep

Following are gadgets with upgraded technology employed for getting sound sleep

(i) Zero sleep coach

It is a fairly new product in the sleep gadget market. It focuses on tracking your sleep patterns in detail but not on waking you up. Zero has in particular attractive web interface. So if you want detailed and thorough sleep records, zero is one way to follow.

(ii). Chillow comfort pillow

These is nothing better than a cold pillow because a hot or humid pillow is annoying. It is a pillow insert that slips inside your pillow case keeping the top of your pillow cold. It is certainly comfortable using soft thermo regulating device to get sound sleep.

(iii) Bed Fan

It lies at the foot of your bed, keeping you cool at night inducing sound sleep.

(iv) Pzizz sleep software

It is a set of audio soundtracks that help you to nap during the day and get to sleep at night.

(v) Light Timer

It is a simple light timer used to turn on lights in your bedroom a 6 minutes before your walk up there by easing you into consciousness.

(vi) Sleep Tractor

It is a device that monitors your sleep cycle via accelerometers.

You can set a window of time during which you want to wake up but it will decide to make you during non-REM sleep so as you wake up easily and look refreshed keeping in view your sleeping pattern and otherwise when you wake up during deep REM sleep then you are completely disoriented and confused.

(vii) Sleep Sound Therapy System
It is also know as sound oasis, being the development of technology in the field of health, is an instrument to facilitate sleep. This unit includes several key features to improve the quality of sleep and help you fall asleep faster, stay asleep longer and sleep ware soundly.

This sound therapy has me feature of relaxation which induces sound sleep and allows users to and new sound by inserting an optional memory card. Basic functions include the enhanced sleep besides fully functioning with backlit brightness digitec alarm clock and calendar variables.

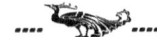

www.ingramcontent.com/pod-product-compliance
Lightning Source LLC
Chambersburg PA
CBHW070335230426
43663CB00011B/2325